prof. dr. heinz-hermann reichenbach-klinke

all about marine aquarium fish diseases

edited by dr. mark p. dulin

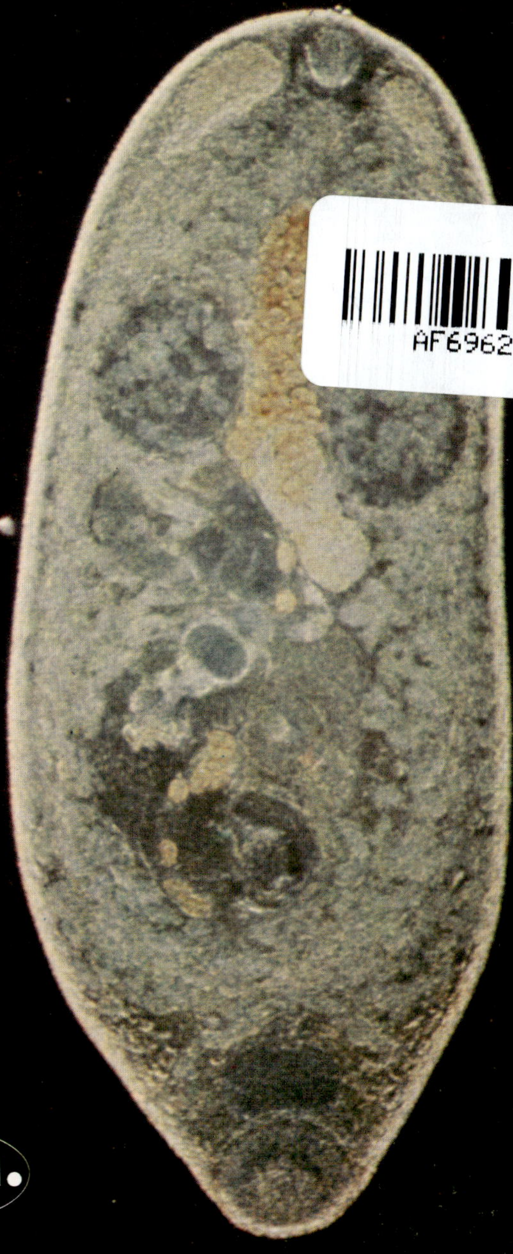

AF696293

t.f.h.

Cover: *Heniochus acuminatus.* Photo by Walt Deas.

Frontispiece: Digenetic fluke. Photo by Frickhinger.

ISBN 0-87666-467-2

©Copyright 1977 by T.F.H. Publications, Inc. Ltd.

Distributed in the U.S.A. by T.F.H. Publications, Inc., 211 West Sylvania Avenue, P.O. Box 27, Neptune City, N.J. 07753; in England by T.F.H. (Gt. Britain) Ltd., 13 Nutley Lane, Reigate, Surrey; in Canada to the book store and library trade by Clarke, Irwin & Company, Clarwin House, 791 St. Clair Avenue West, Toronto 10, Ontario; in Canada to the pet trade by Rolf C. Hagen Ltd., 3225 Sartelon Street, Montreal 382, Quebec; in Southeast Asia by Y.W. Ong, 9 Lorong 36 Geylang, Singapore 14; in Australia and the south Pacific by Pet Imports Pty. Ltd., P.O. Box 149, Brookvale 2100, N.S.W., Australia. Published by T.F.H. Publications Inc. Ltd., The British Crown Colony of Hong Kong.

Contents

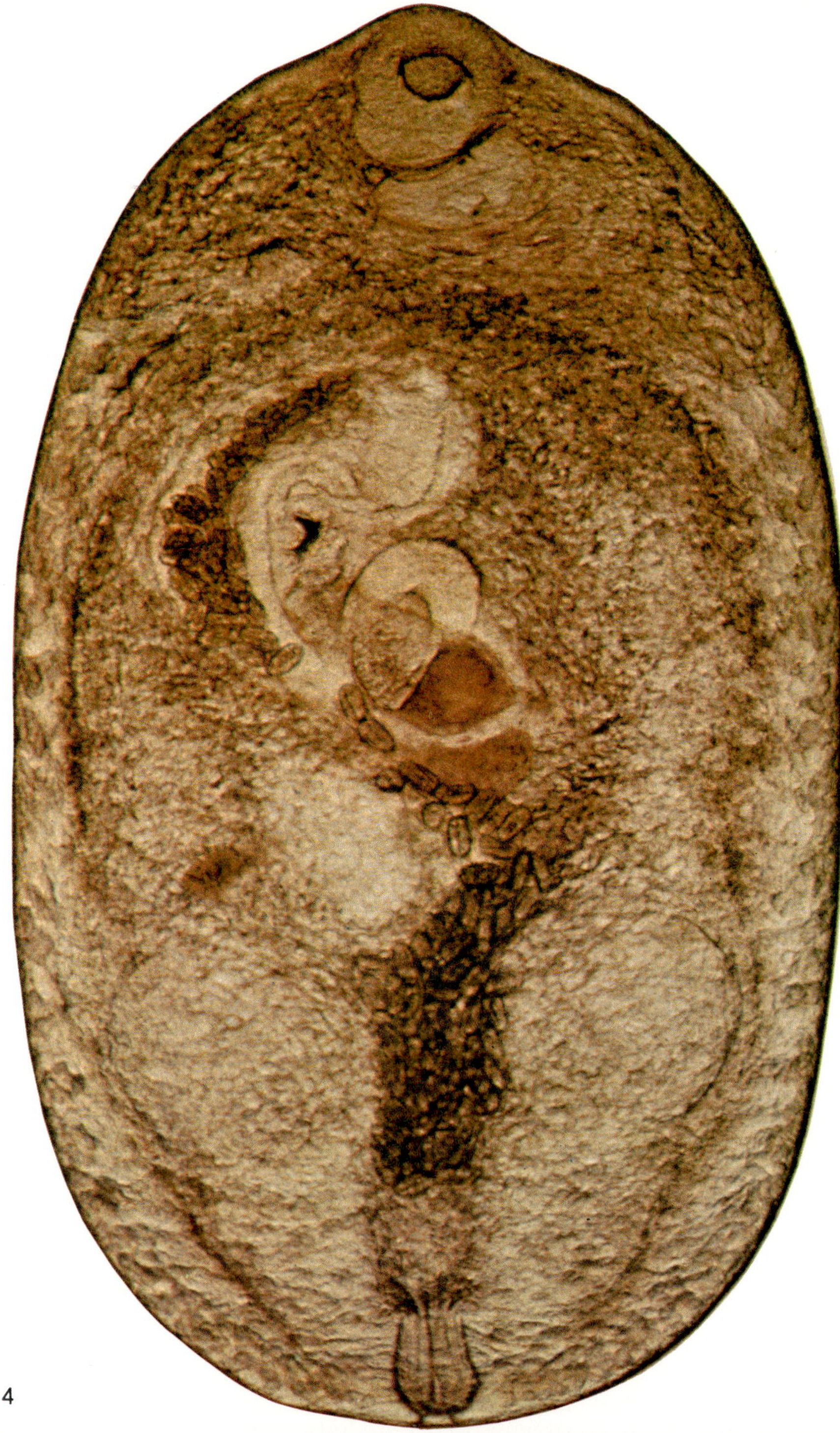

4

Preface

Marine fish diagnostic and treatment procedures are still in their infancy. Although information is published in specialized scientific journals, there are very few books that have been devoted to diseases of marine fishes. Many times the information which is published is too specialized to suit the needs of aquarists and distributors of marine fishes. It therefore appears that a contribution toward protecting marine aquarium fishes would be valuable. It is hoped that the information presented here will serve the needs of both the scientific community and the marine hobbyist.

Prof. Dr. H.-H. Reichenbach-Klinke

These digenetic flukes (frontispiece, opposite page, and below) were all recovered from the intestinal tracts of marine fishes. Photos by Frickhinger.

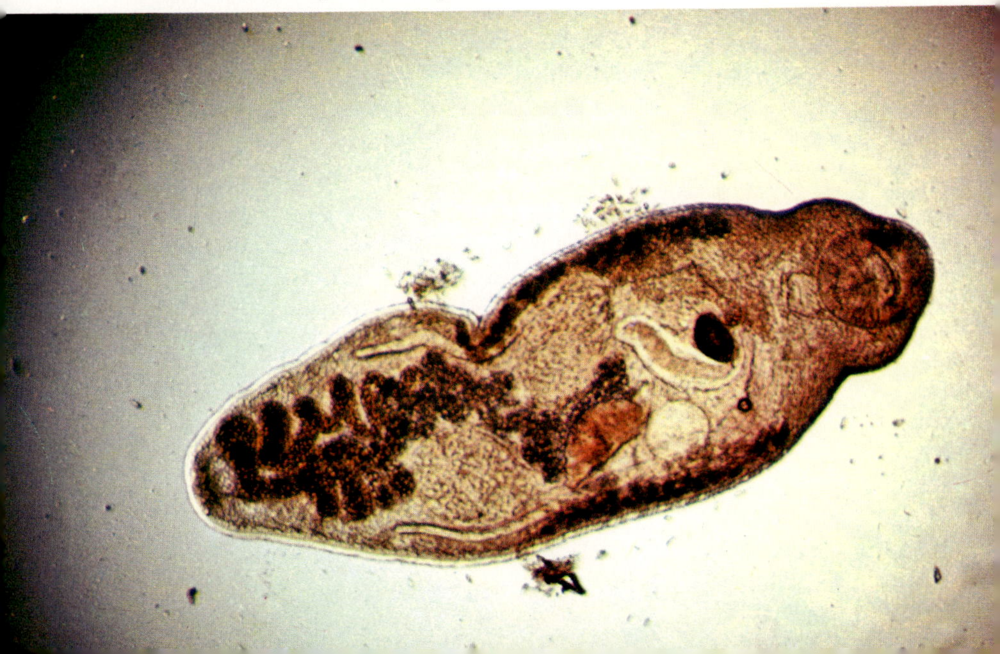

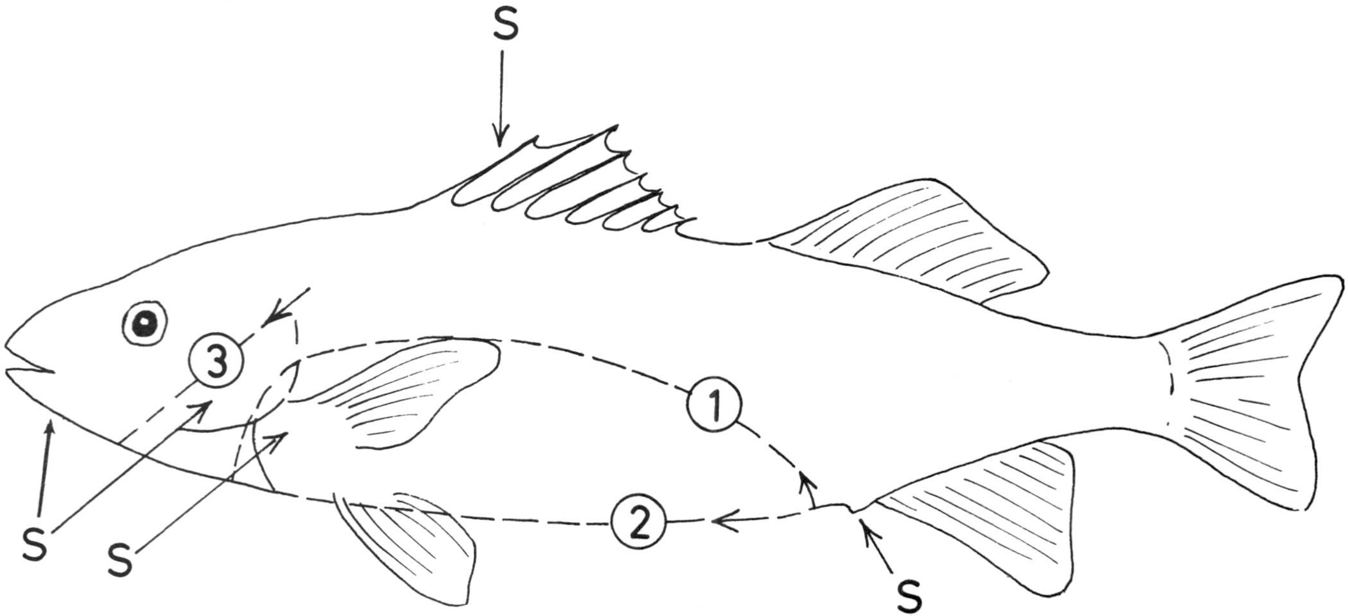

INCISION LINES FOR DISSECTING A FISH

When making the incisions (1,2) to reveal the internal tissues, be careful not to puncture the intestinal tract. By removing the operculum (3) the gills can be studied. Imprint smears (S) should be made from various body surfaces, the gills and any external lesions.

I. Inspection, Investigation and Painless Killing of Diseased Fishes

The marine aquarium must be inspected daily so that any abnormalities that develop can be discovered in the early stages. The fishes should be carefully observed for any abnormal movements, changes in eating behavior or respiratory difficulty. Water quality parameters also should be carefully monitored to assure provision of a proper environment for the captive species.

Investigations conducted on diseased fishes must be done very carefully, as most fishes are quite sensitive to touch. Care must be taken not to damage the skin or cause the loss of scales. It is often advisable to use an anesthetic to avoid further stressing an already sick fish and to protect the diagnostician from injury while handling venomous fishes such as the lionfishes (*Pterois*, *Dendrochirus*, etc., spp.). Imprint smears should be made from external lesions as well as from the base of fins, about the anus and from the gills. If no abnormalities are detected from the external examination of the fish and pathogenic organisms are not detected from stained and unstained imprint smears, it must be assumed that the fish is suffering from internal damage.

In certain instances the diagnostician may elect to sacrifice a diseased specimen in hopes of obtaining a diagnosis that might reduce future losses. The killing of the fish must be as painless as possible. A small fish can

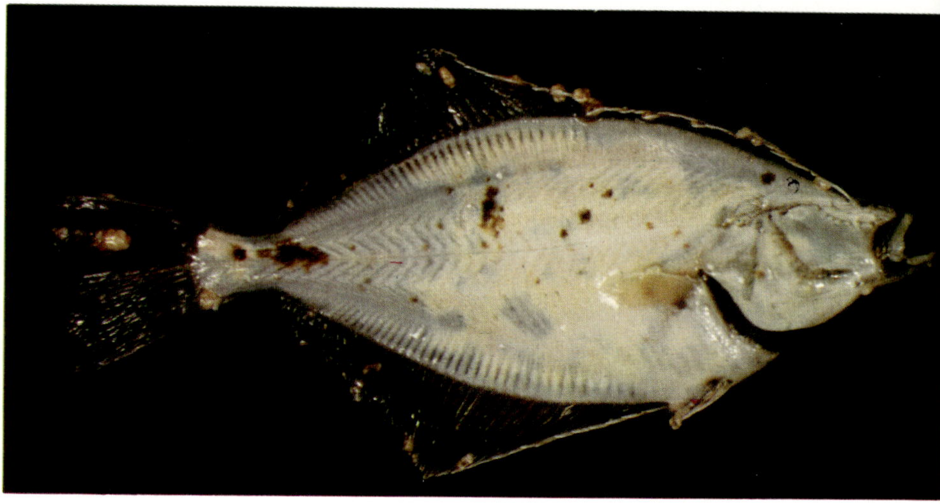

This fish is suffering from lymphocystis; the virus responsible for this disease grows within connective tissue cells of the skin. Notice that the hypertrophied fibroblasts which contain this virus (below) are surrounded by a hyaline capsule.

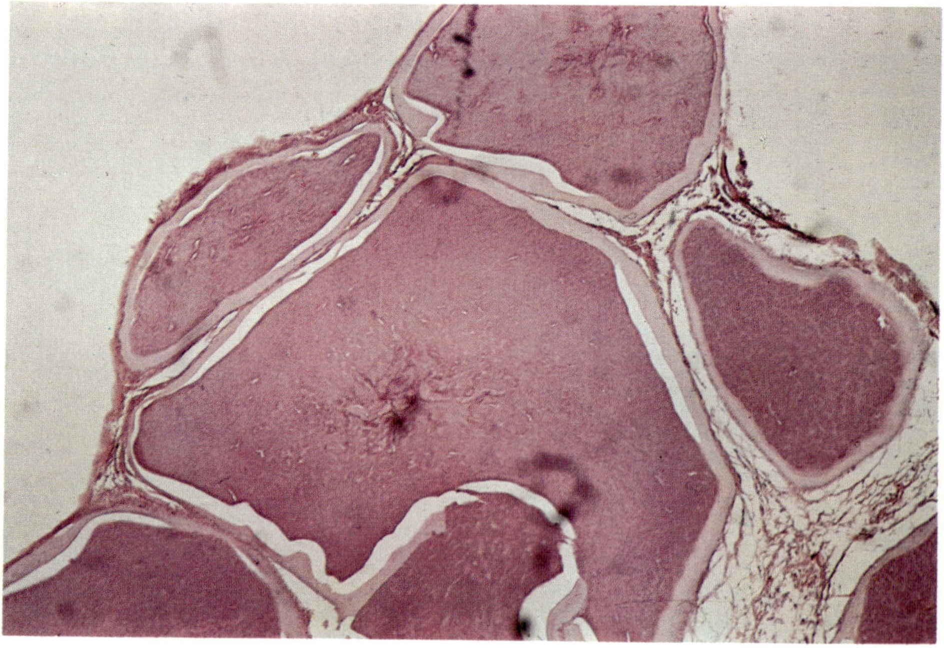

be humanely killed by making a quick severance of the spinal cord, just behind the head. Larger fishes should be anesthetized prior to severing the spinal cord. One of the commonly used fish anesthetics is tricaine methanesulfonate (MS-222), manufactured by Sandoz Pharmaceuticals, Hanover, New Jersey and distributed in small quantities by Ayerst Laboratories as Finquel.® Dosages vary from 1:1,000 to 1:20,000 according to the sensitivity of the fish. Medium-size fishes are narcotized within a few minutes when a 1:2,000 to 1:3,000 solution is used. The drug can either be mixed with the water in which the fish is contained or squirted into the mouth or gill cavity.

The instruments required for a post-mortem examination are very minimal. If a scalpel, scissors and forceps are not readily available, a single-edged razor blade, manicure scissors and tweezers will suffice.

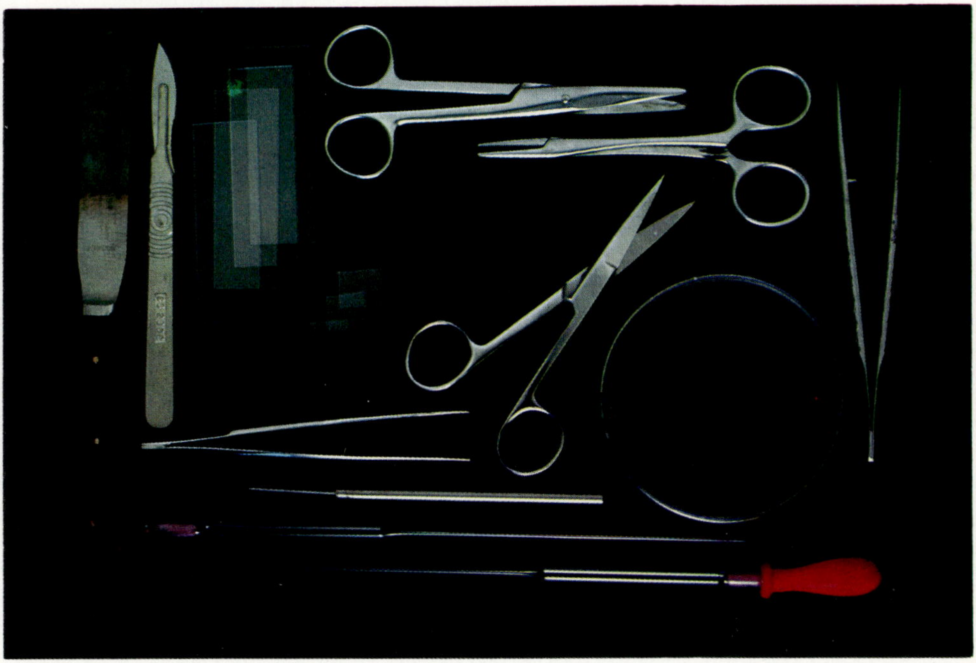

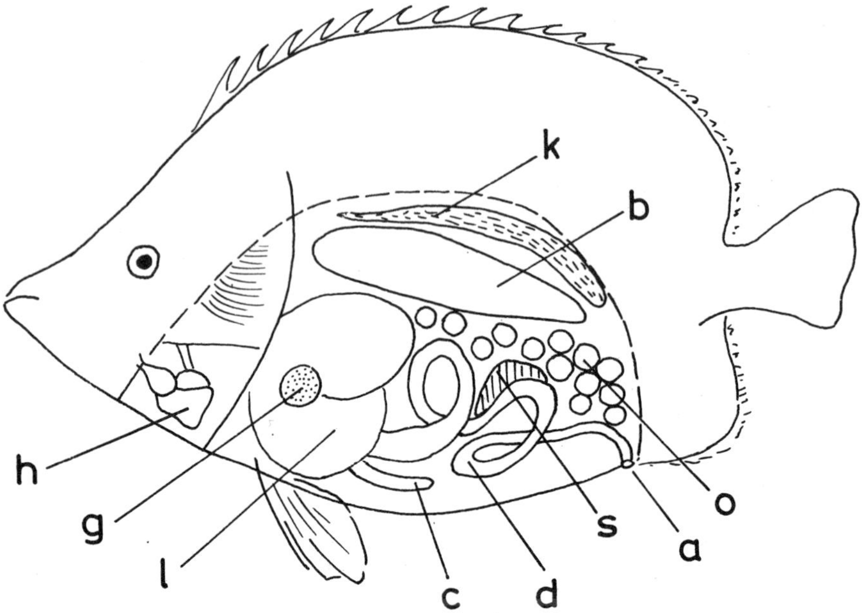

This schematic drawing of a dissected fish reveals the: a. anus, b. swimbladder, c. caecum, d. intestine, g. gall bladder, h. heart, k. kidney, l. liver, o. ovary, and s. spleen.

Chlorobutanol (1,1,1 trichlor-2-methyl-2-propanol) is also used as a fish anesthetic. When the fish is placed in a solution containing 1 g/liter, anesthesia occurs within 40 seconds and lasts for 6 to 8 minutes. Another fish anesthetic is 2-methylquinoline (Quinaldine® Eastman Kodak Co., Rochester, N.Y.). The dosage of the solution is 5 to 12 ppm.

Once the fish has been properly dissected, blood smears can be made from the heart blood. A smear also should be made from the intestinal contents, and imprints should be made from the liver, kidney, ovaries or testes and occasionally from muscles and brain. These smears should be stained and microscopically examined for the presence of pathological changes or pathogenic organisms.

II. Infectious Diseases

VIRUSES

The most common viral disease of marine fishes is lymphocystis virus. It was first described from the European flounder *Pleuronectes flesus.* It has since been reported from a variety of both freshwater and saltwater fishes (2, 26). Lymphocystis disease is characterized by dermal papillomas that usually occur on the dorsal fin but may also occur on the tail fin as well as the body surface.

Lymphocystic cells are hypertrophied fibroblasts. The connective tissue cells can enlarge to enormous size (340 microns) and are surrounded by a hyaline capsule. Intracytoplasmic inclusions give a positive Feulgen reaction. The disease has been successfully transmitted using ultracentrifugates and bacteria-free filtrates. Lymphocystis disease occurs in both natural populations and in aquariums. Wild populations have had up to 1% incidence; in aquarium populations, this of course can be more. Polluted water is suspected of predisposing fishes to acquiring this disease. The exact mechanism of transmission is not known; some species appear to have a natural resistance. There is no known course of therapy for this disease.

Other hyperplastic diseases suspected of having a viral etiology include "papilloma" disease of flatfish and "cauliflower" disease of eels (Stomato-papillomatosis).

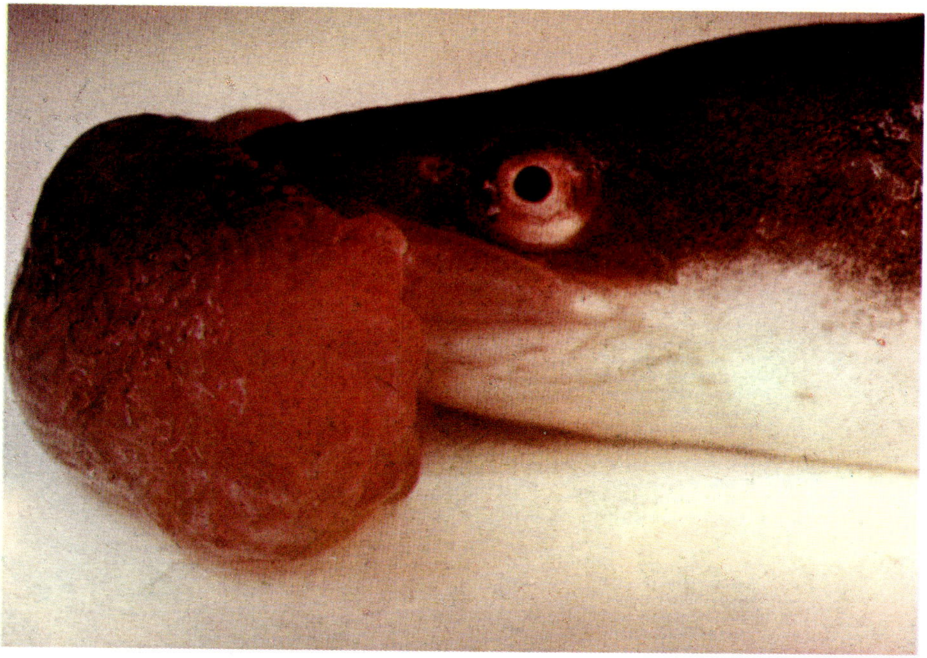

Stomato-papillomatosis ("cauliflower" disease) of eels is a contagious disease thought to be caused by a virus. The papillomatous growth on the caudal peduncle of the fish below was also thought to be caused by a virus. Photos by Frickhinger.

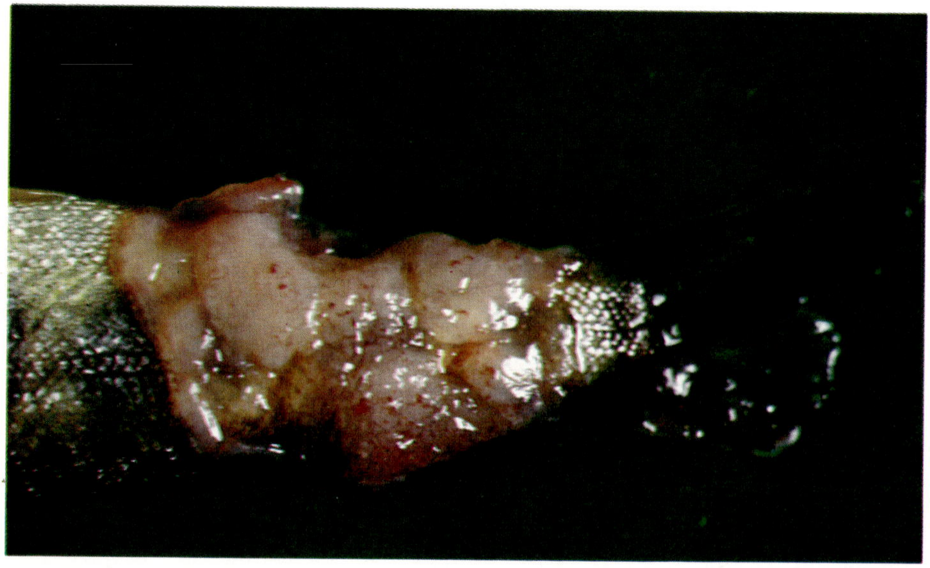

Equipped with powerful suckers for attachment, digenetic flukes can damage the fish's intestinal mucosa. Large numbers of these parasites can debilitate the host.

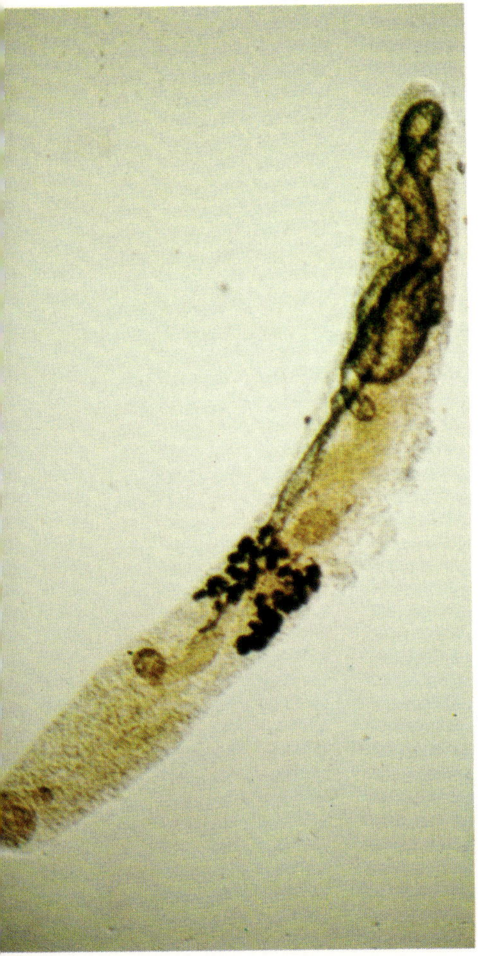

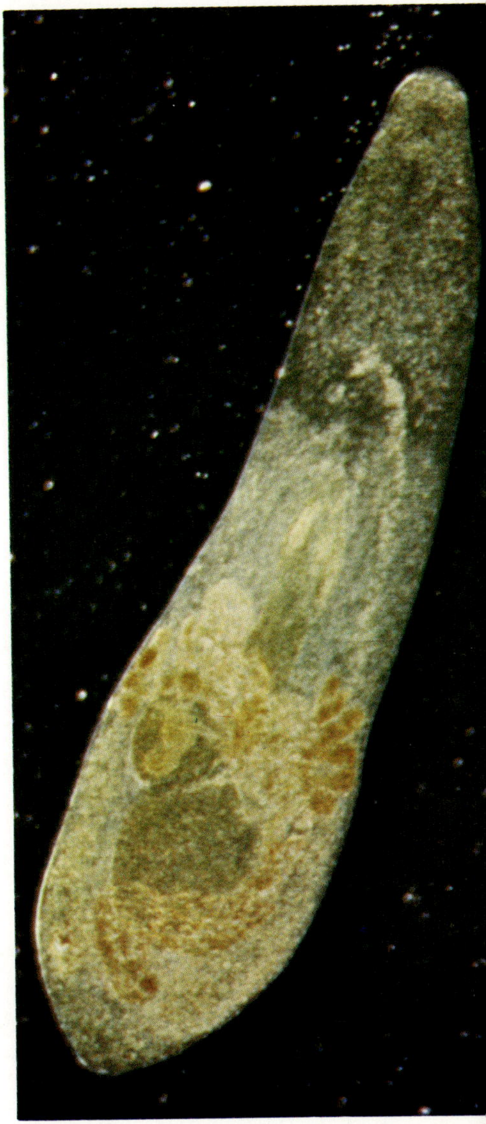

Both of these digenetic flukes were isolated from the intestines of a *Chaetodon leucopleura.* Photos by Frickhinger.

This disease is characterized by cauliflower-like growths that usually occur in the jaw area. These hypertrophied areas are reddish-white or brownish and consist of narrowly folded dermal cells. Sometimes islands of degenerative cells occur in the dermal layer, isolated from the normal epithelial cells.

Large papillomatous growths on the jaws of eels interfere with feeding, so an emaciated condition frequently occurs. Losses are especially heavy among young eels. The disease is contagious and appears to be seasonal in that the incidence is low in spring and autumn. Maximum size of the growth occurs in August and September (41). A correlation may exist between the water temperature and dissolved oxygen level and the severity of the infection. Although a proved course of therapy is unknown, limited data suggest that quinine sulfate therapy may be beneficial (42).

Parasitic ciliates (*Miamiensis avidus*) are suspected of transmitting a tumor-like disease to the seahorse *Hippocampus erectus* (32). Experimental evidence suggests that infectious pancreatic necrosis (IPN) virus can be transmitted to marine fishes (*Haemulon sciurus*), as live cell cultures died after the inoculation of IPN virus (33). Using this same *Haemulon sciurus* cell line, other researchers found a presumed "orphan virus" which was destructive to primary explants and fish cell lines (9).

Investigators are still in the early stages of marine fish virology. Three viral diseases (lymphocystis, cauliflower disease of eels, and IPN) are currently known to infect marine fishes; several other viruses are suspected of infecting marine fishes. A few years ago only 5 viruses were known to infect freshwater fishes; today over 15 freshwater viral agents have been discovered. It is probable that further investigations will demonstrate many more viruses that are pathogenic to marine fishes.

BACTERIA

Bacterial diseases commonly affect marine fishes, and it is presumed that most losses among marine aquarium fishes are caused by this group of organisms.

Aeromonas and *Pseudomonas* bacteria commonly occur in both the freshwater and saltwater environments. Pathogenic aeromonads and pseudomonads cause a variety of clinical signs of disease, including dermal ulcerations, reddening and inflammation. *Pseudomonas* (syn. *Aeromobacter*) *ichthyodermis* is responsible for causing infectious dermatitis of certain marine fishes (68).

Bacterial fin- and tail-rot also occurs in marine fishes. Several pathogenic bacteria, including aeromonads, pseudomonads and myxobacteria, are responsible for this condition. Columnaris disease, caused by the myxobacterium *Flexibacter* (syn. *Chondrococcus*) *columnaris*, is often resistant to antibacterial therapy. Some antibiotics that have been successfully used are kanamycin at 20 mg/kg (11), or either chloramphenicol or Aureomycin® at the rate of 10-20 ppm in the aquarium water. A 10- to 15-minute bath in a hydrogen peroxide solution (20 ml of commercial 3% solution in one liter of water) has also reportedly been successful (13). Other agents used to treat gill necrosis associated with columnaris include oxytetracycline, nifurpirinol and copper sulfate.

One of the most common bacterial diseases of marine fishes is vibriosis, also known as boil or ulcer disease. *Vibrio anguillarum*, *V. parahemolyticus* and *V. alginolyticus* have been responsible for extensive mortalities among eels, cod, plaice and herring. The disease is worldwide in distribution. Because all marine fishes are considered susceptible (60), the disease undoubtedly also occurs in the marine aquarium. Vibriosis has been successfully treated with various sulfonamides, nitrofurans and oxytetracycline.

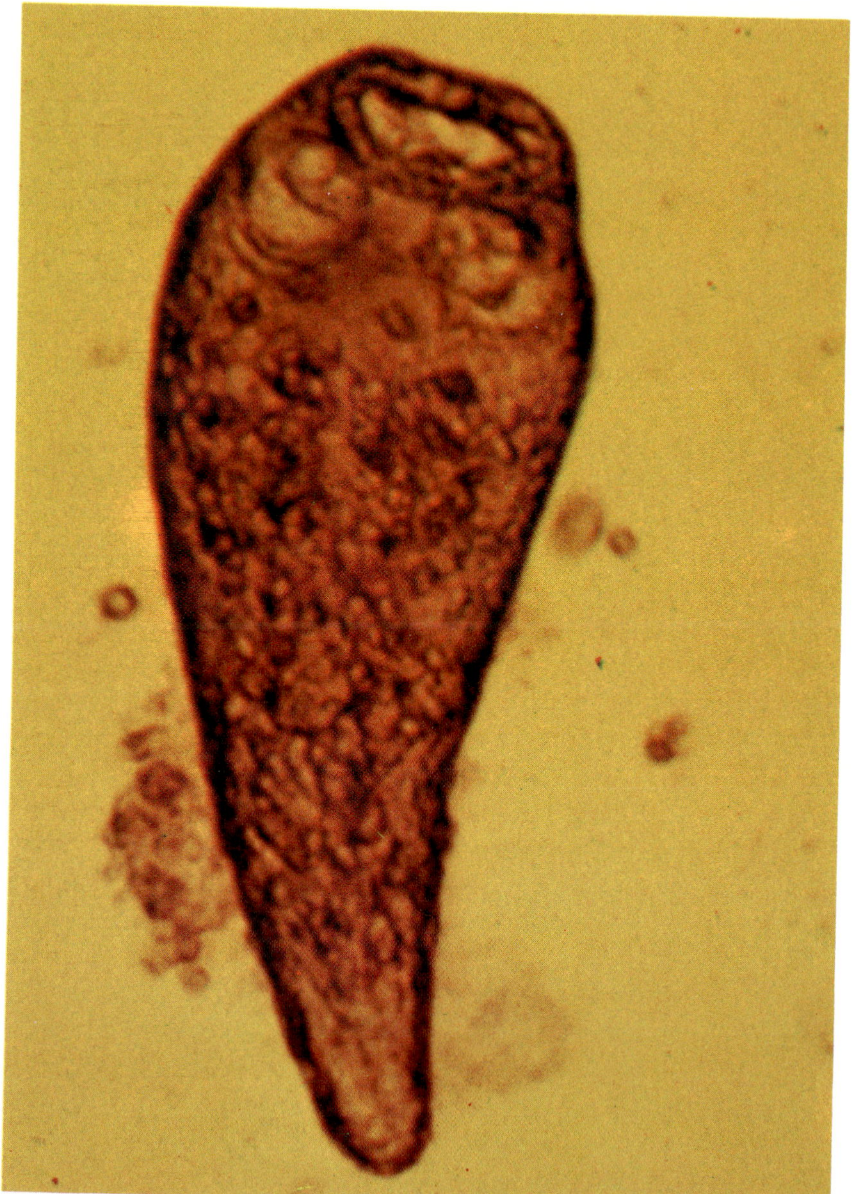

The intermediate larval stages (metacercaria) of tapeworm development have been found beneath the skin, within various internal organs, even within the fish's eye! It is these larval forms which are associated with the most damage to infected fish. Photo by Frickhinger.

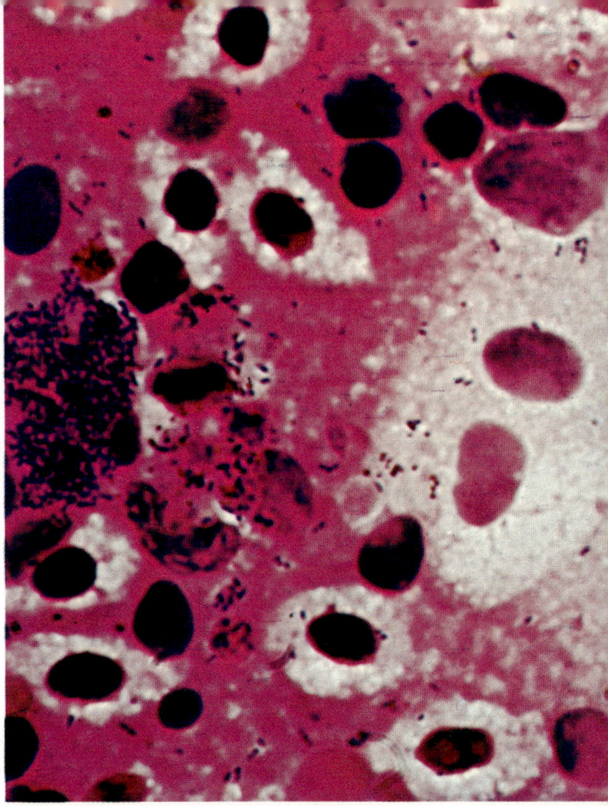

Kidney disease, caused by a Gram-positive *Corynebacterium* sp., is a serious pathogen of freshwater fishes. These diplobacilli were also suspected of being the primary cause of the hypertrophied kidney in the *Thalassoma pavo* shown below. Photo below by Frickhinger.

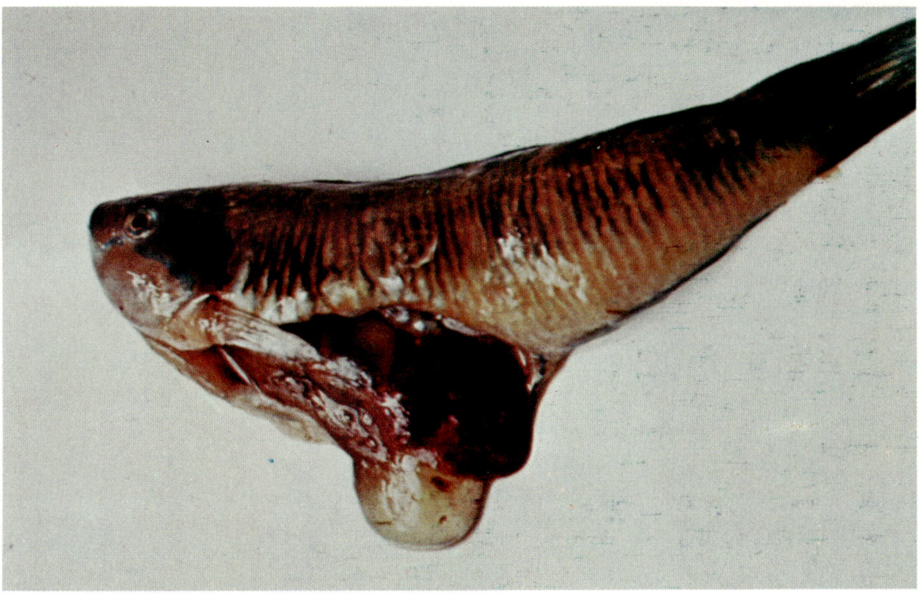

Bacterial kidney disease, also known as Dee disease, is caused by members of the genus *Corynebacterium*. External clinical signs of disease are often not apparent; petechial hemorrhages may occur on the skin, and exophthalmos can occur. Internally, the kidney becomes swollen and affected with whitish lesions.

Anaerobic bacteria were recently found to be pathogenic to various marine fishes (*Mugil cephalus, Sciaenops ocellata, Arius felis*). A *Catenabacterium* was isolated from the blood, liver, kidney and brain of these diseased fishes. Affected fishes were disoriented and weak, and they swam at the surface of the water. This anaerobic pathogen was resistant to gentamycin, kanamycin, neomycin, penicillin G, and polymyxin B. Only chloramphenicol, erythromycin and tetracycline were reported effective (18). Another rare bacterial disease of marine fishes reportedly involved an infection of seahorses (*Hippocampus* spp.) with *Streptothrix* sp. (8).

The bacterial disease most commonly reported in marine aquarium fishes is tuberculosis, caused by *Mycobacterium marinum.* Other pathogenic species of mycobacteria (*M. piscium* and *M. fortuitum*) have also been reported.

The clinical signs of mycobacteriosis vary greatly. Dermatitis, loss of normal coloration, scale defects and loss of scales, fin destruction, exophthalmia and deformities of the jaw and vertebrae have all been reported. Internally, whitish nodules are seen in the liver, kidney and spleen; they are rarely seen in the heart, gills, musculature, eyes, brain and gonads. Acid-fast bacilli may be recovered from all the affected organs and tissues; however, the causative organism is seldom found in older granulomatous nodules.

Stress is thought to play a major role in predisposing fishes to acquiring tuberculosis. Adverse water quality, insufficient illumination, poor nutrition and inadequate levels of dissolved oxygen increase the fishes' susceptibility to this disease. Because amphibians and reptiles can also have tuberculosis, they serve as potential sources of infection.

Human infections associated with tuberculosis of aquarium fishes have been reported. These rare occurrences are generally localized and limited to skin lesions. *M. fortuitum* is capable of growth at 37° C and is most commonly incriminated in human lesions that have been acquired from diseased fishes. Human infections with *M. marinum* have not been confirmed, yet they cannot be denied, as the organism is closely related to the human pathogen *M. kansasi*.

Exophthalmia (popeye) can be caused by a variety of infectious diseases including bacterial kidney disease and piscine tuberculosis. This squirrelfish (*Adioryx* sp.) is receiving an antibacterial injection in hopes of arresting the condition.

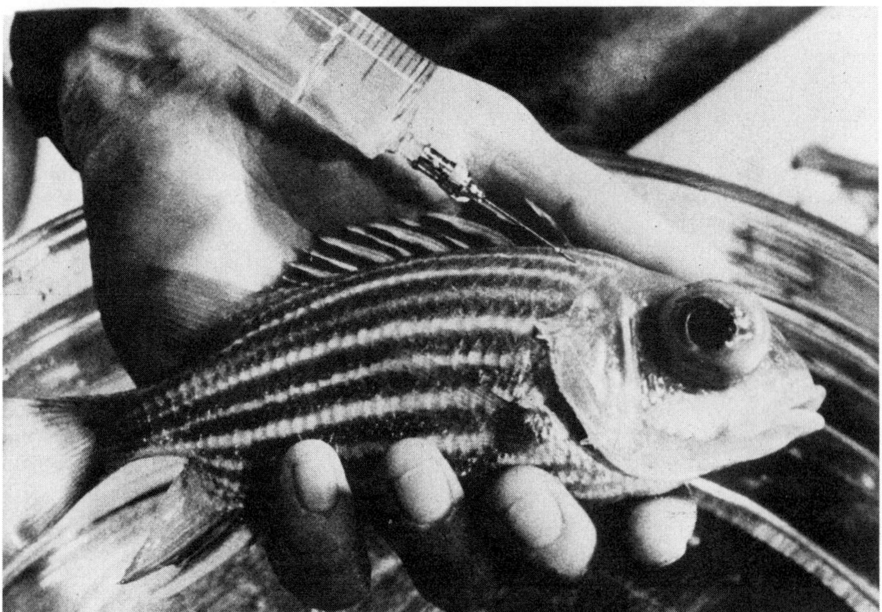

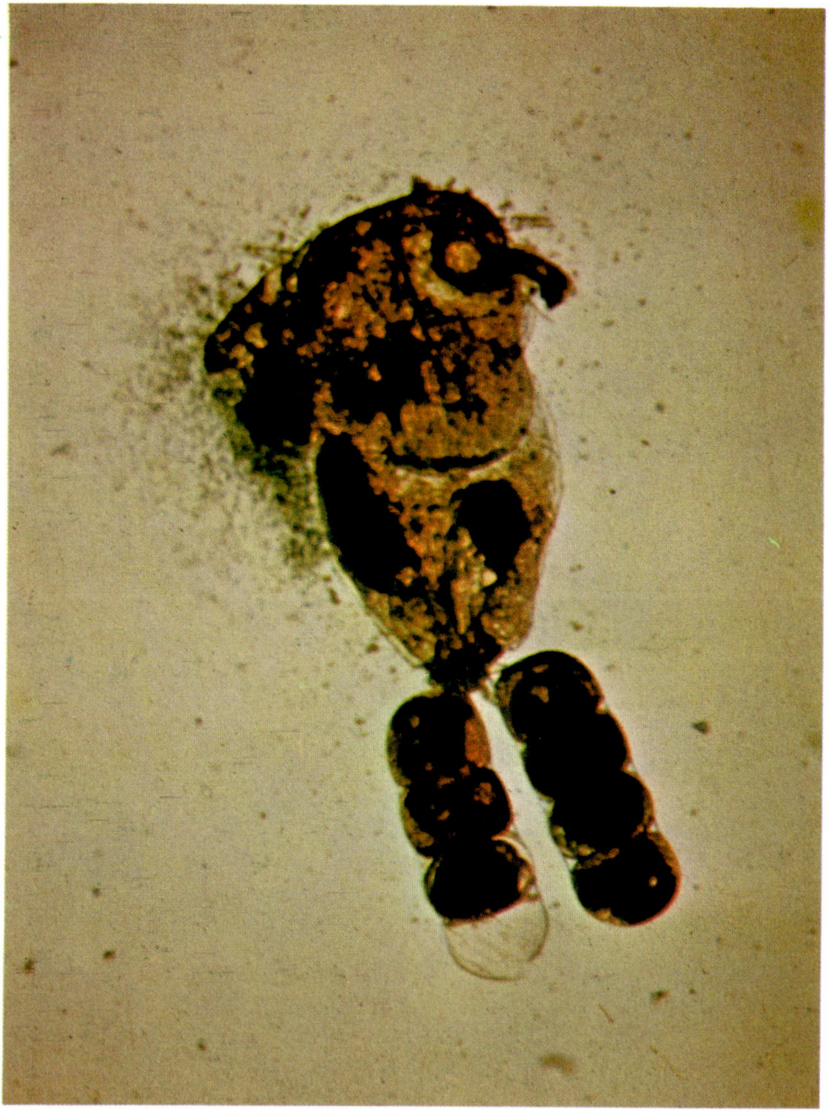

Parasitic copepods such as this *Lamproglena* sp. can seriously damage the gills of marine fishes. Small numbers of these parasites can be carefully removed from the gills or skin with forceps. Heavy infestations are best treated with a series of Dylox® (Masoten®) baths. Photo by Frickhinger.

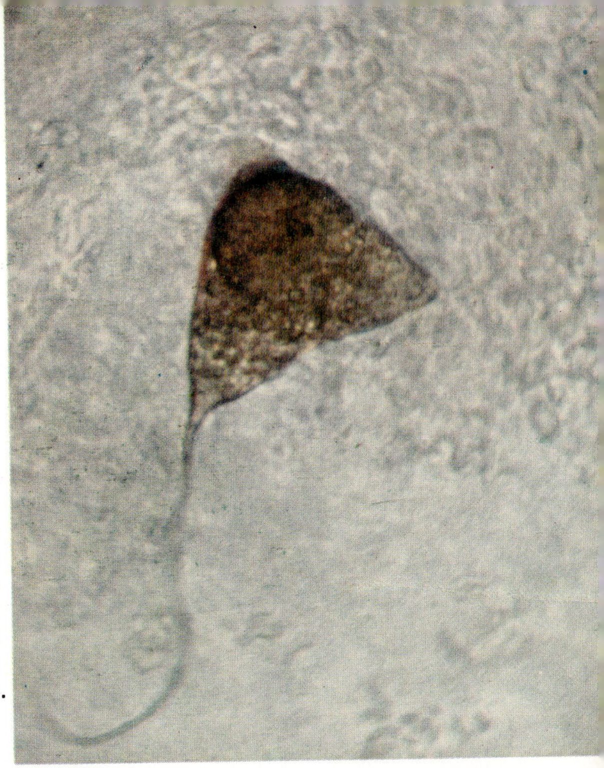

Monogenetic flukes in the genus *Trochopus* commonly inhabit the gills of searobins (Triglidae). The pyramidal egg (right) with a long attachment filament is characteristic.

This fluke (*Accacoelium* sp.) was found parasitizing *Heniochus permutatus.* Photo by Frickhinger.

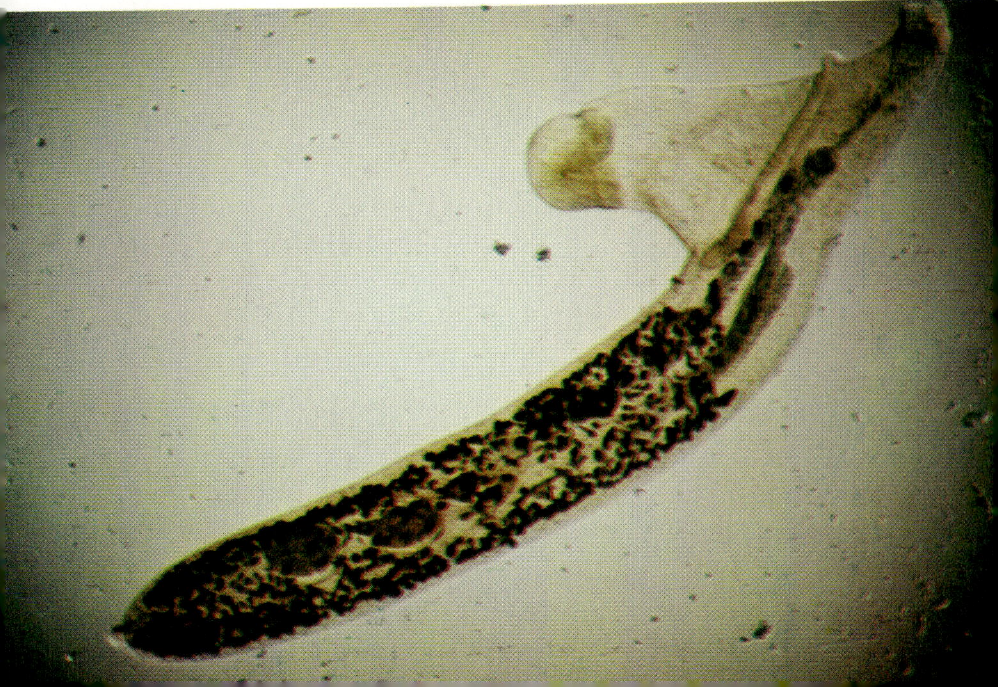

Limited success has been obtained by treating piscine tuberculosis with antibiotics. Both kanamycin- and tetracycline-impregnated foods have been used. Because the disease affects mostly weakened animals, prevention is of greater importance than treatment.

To date, relatively little is known about bacterial diseases of tropical marine aquarium fishes; future investigations will undoubtedly reveal many more pathogenic species. Generally speaking, marine fishes have a high degree of immunocompetence; therefore, preventing bacterial infections with specific immunizing agents is a distinct possibility. In the meantime, most bacterial infections can be successfully treated with antibiotics. Caution should be exercised when using these drugs, because the development of drug-resistant strains of bacteria may occur.

Because of poor vascularization in the fish's musculature, intramuscular injections are not recommended. Injectables should either be given in the dorsal commissure (nape) or intraperitoneally.

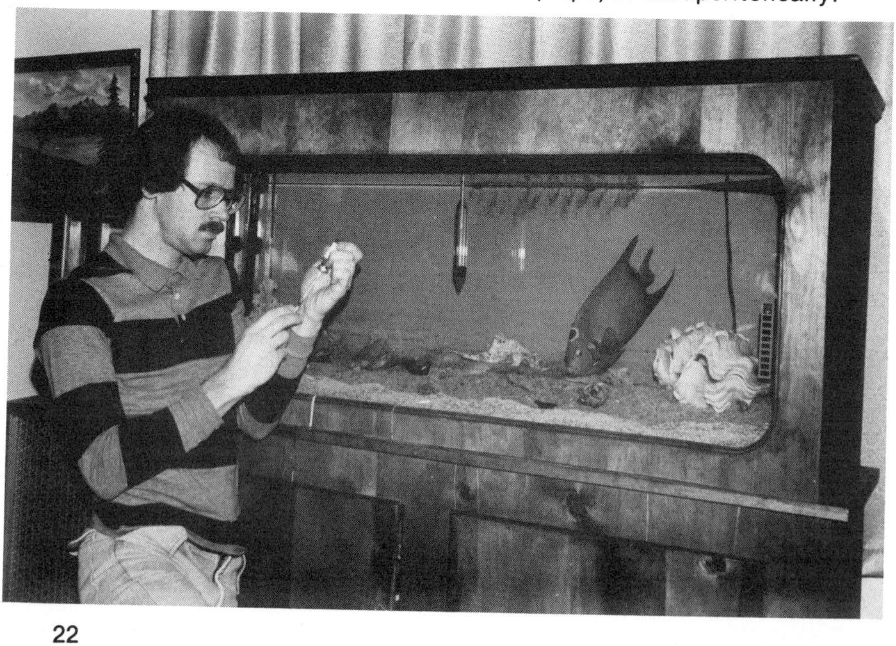

FUNGI

The most commonly described mycosis of marine aquarium fishes is *Ichthyophonus* (syn. *Ichthyosporidium*) infection. Systemic infections involving *Ichthyophonus hoferi* occur in both the natural environment and in aquariums.

Clinical signs of *Ichthyophonus* infection include loss of appetite, emaciation, discoloration, damaged skin and fins, exophthalmos and (rarely) cases of dermatitis. Internal lesions include nodules in the musculature, liver, spleen, heart, brain, stomach and intestines. These nodules are composed of the fungal plasmodium and are encapsulated by the host's tissue. Both elements continue to grow until the parasite escapes from the cyst. The parasitic fungus develops branches with swollen tips; new nodules may form at these tips. Within the fungal plasmodia, spores that can spread out to infect other tissues develop. The initial infection begins with the uptake of fungal material; the cyst walls are dissolved by the gastro-intestinal juices, allowing the infective fungus to penetrate the intestinal wall. Once it becomes systemic, the fungus spreads to various body organs and tissues via the circulatory system. When established in a particular tissue, the organism can spread from the maternal organism to produce new nodules.

Marine fishes infected with *Ichthyophonus* commonly have germinating plasmodial material contained within broad hyphae. If only cysts occur, the pathological changes could be confused with those of piscine tuberculosis. A tentative differential diagnosis is based upon stained tissue imprints. A definitive diagnosis of *Ichthyophonus hoferi* infection is based upon culturing infectious material upon Sabouraud's medium. When *Ichthyophonus* germinates on an artificial medium, "daughter-balls" are formed.

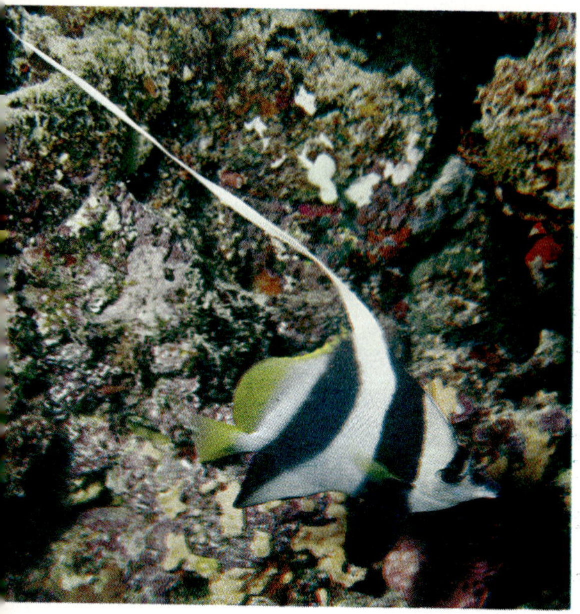

This beautiful *Heniochus acuminatus* is in a perfect state of health. Contrastingly, the *Heniochus acuminatus* shown below is diseased. Coloration and fin integrity give valuable clues in the recognition of diseased fish. Above photo by Allan Power. Photo below by Dr. Shih-chieh Shen.

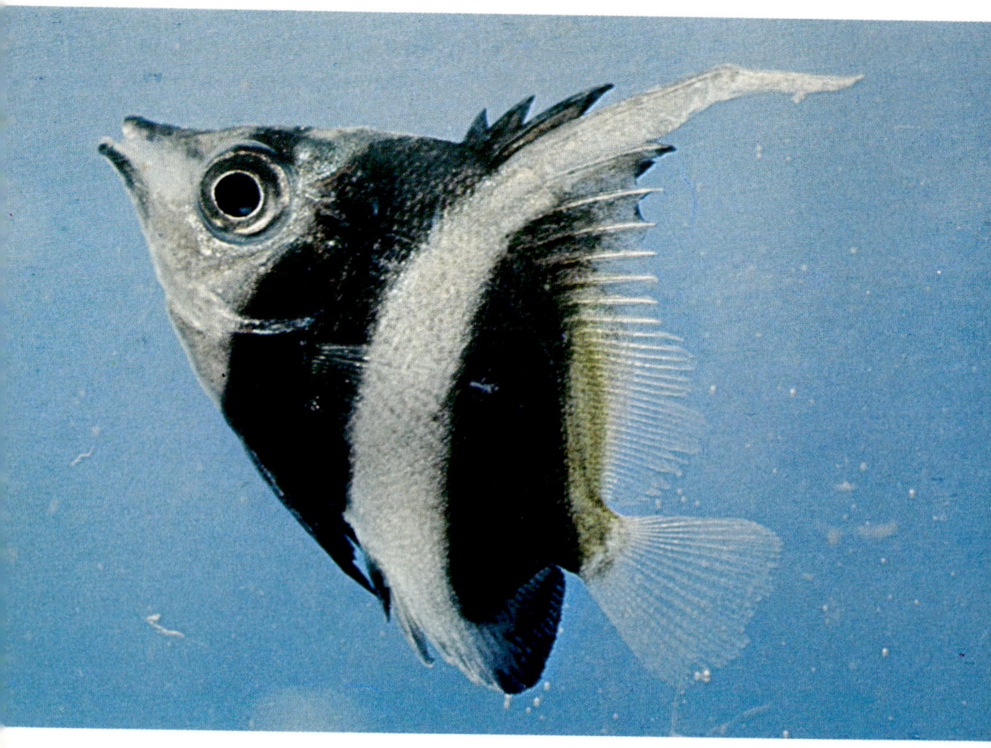

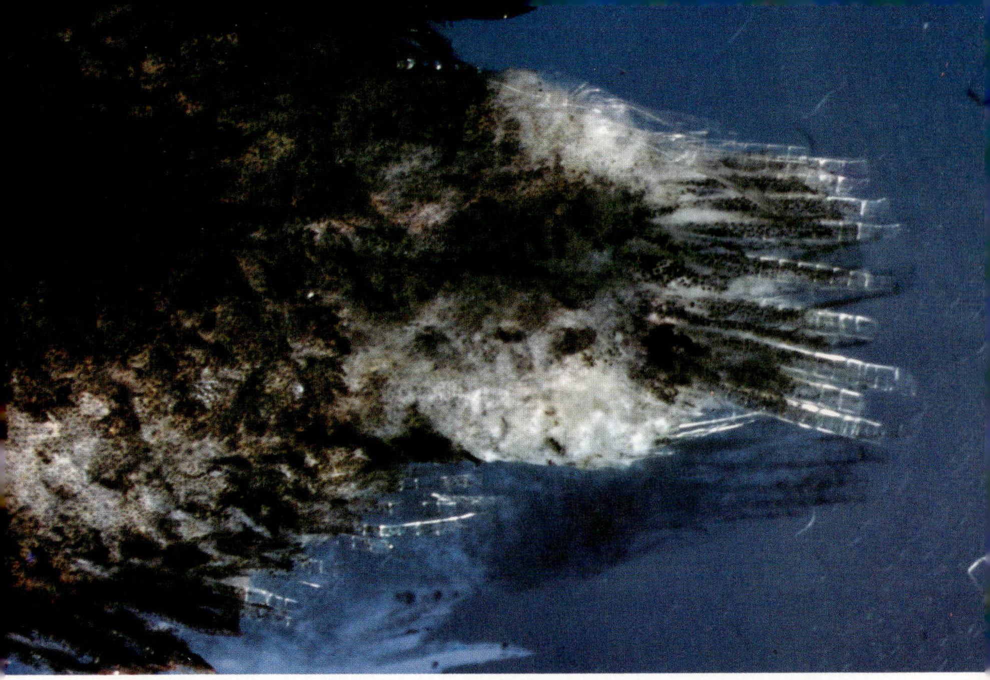

When bacteria cause erosion and cell death, as in tail rot, *Saprolegnia* commonly invades the necrotic tissue. After a proper period of antibiotic therapy this caudal fin should regenerate.

When a fish dies of a suspected bacterial disease, prompt examination of the blood may reveal systemic bacteria. Several rod-shaped bacteria (arrow) can be seen here. Photomicrograph courtesy Piscisan Ltd.

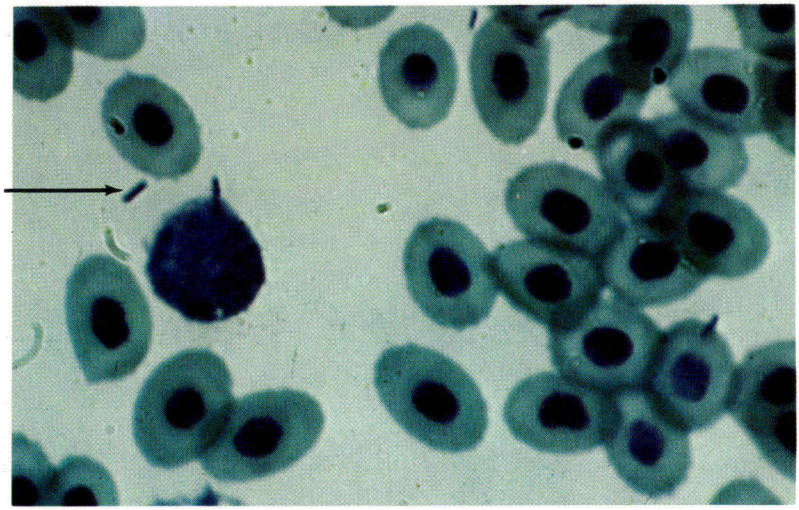

There is no known treatment for *Ichthyophonus* infections of fishes. The pathogen can be introduced via unprocessed fish flesh so caution must be exercised when feeding raw food products. Maintaining good environmental conditions in the aquarium, coupled with supplemental vitamin therapy, can increase the fishes' resistance to diseases.

Several fungi are known to attack the external surface of fishes in the marine environment. One of the most common fungal parasites that occurs in both fresh and salt water is *Saprolegnia*. This fungus acts only as a secondary opportunistic pathogen, attacking the weakened or wounded fish whose skin is damaged by mechanical or chemical disturbances. *Isoachlya parasitica*, another member of the family Saprolegniaceae, was reported infecting *Atherina siqueti* in Southern France (1).

Treatment of external fungal infections can be accomplished by painting the affected areas with a 10% povidone-iodine solution or giving the fish a bath in an antifungal solution. Some of the treatments that have been used include a 30- to 90-minute bath in a potassium permanganate solution (1 g potassium permanganate in 100 liters of water) or a 10- to 30-minute copper sulfate bath (5 to 10 g of copper sulfate per 100 liters of water). Since *Saprolegnia* is a secondary invader, long-term success can be obtained only if the primary cause of the weakened skin condition also is alleviated.

Isolated reports of rare mycotic infections of marine fishes include a liver infection in a ray (*Trygon pastinaceae*) by a fungus closely related to *Pullularia*. Fungi have also been reported in the ray's teeth. Parasitic fungi were also found in sharks and in hypertrophied gill filaments of the cod (*Gadus morhua*).

With the exception of *Ichthyophonus* infections,

knowledge of parasitic fungi of marine fishes is rather scant. Further reports of fungal infections involving marine aquarium fishes are expected in the near future.

ALGAE

Rare, isolated cases of parasitic algae causing disease in marine fishes were reported in the 1930's. A parasitic member of the Cyanophycea, *Anacamptothrix intestinalis*, was reported in the intestines of the marine fish *Mugil chelo*. Two other algal pathogens, *Leucosphaera oxneri* and *Thalamoebella parasitica*, were incriminated in causing an epizootic and mortalities in the Monaco Oceanarium (44).

Fishes in a marine aquarium can be killed as a result of an overabundance of algae just as oceanic fish-kills occasionally occur as a result of excessive algal growth. Photo by Dr. Herbert R. Axelrod.

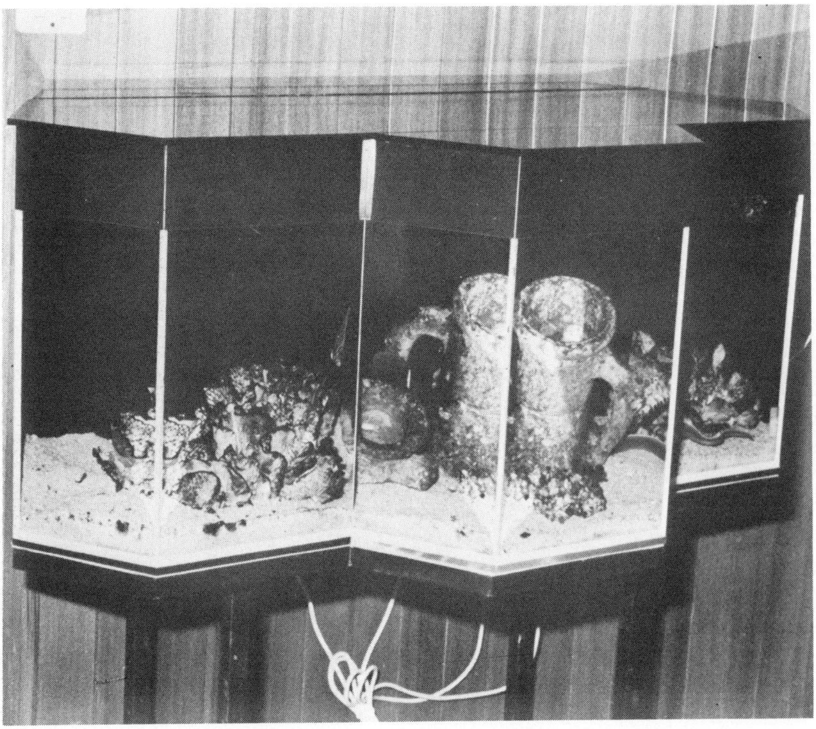

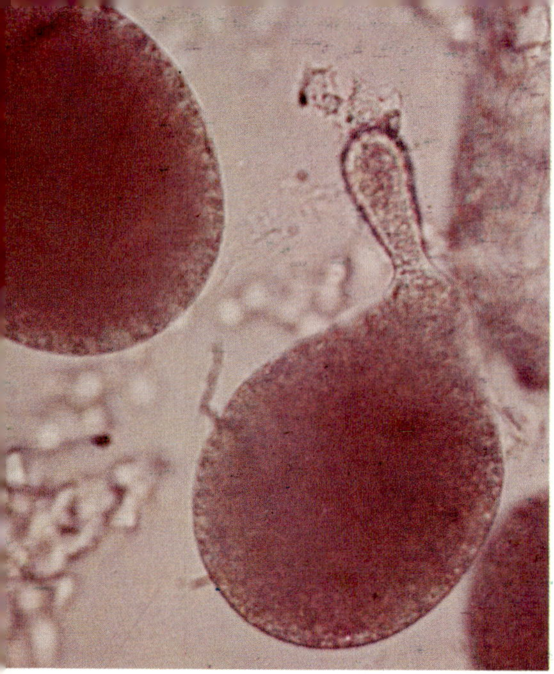

Left: Sporulation of the fungus *Ichthyophonus hoferi* occurs both within fish tissue and after a suitable incubation time on Sabouraud's medium. Photo by Glenn L. Hoffman. **Below:** A *Toxotes* is heavily parasitized by an external fungus, most likely a species of *Saprolegnia.* Photo by Frickhinger.

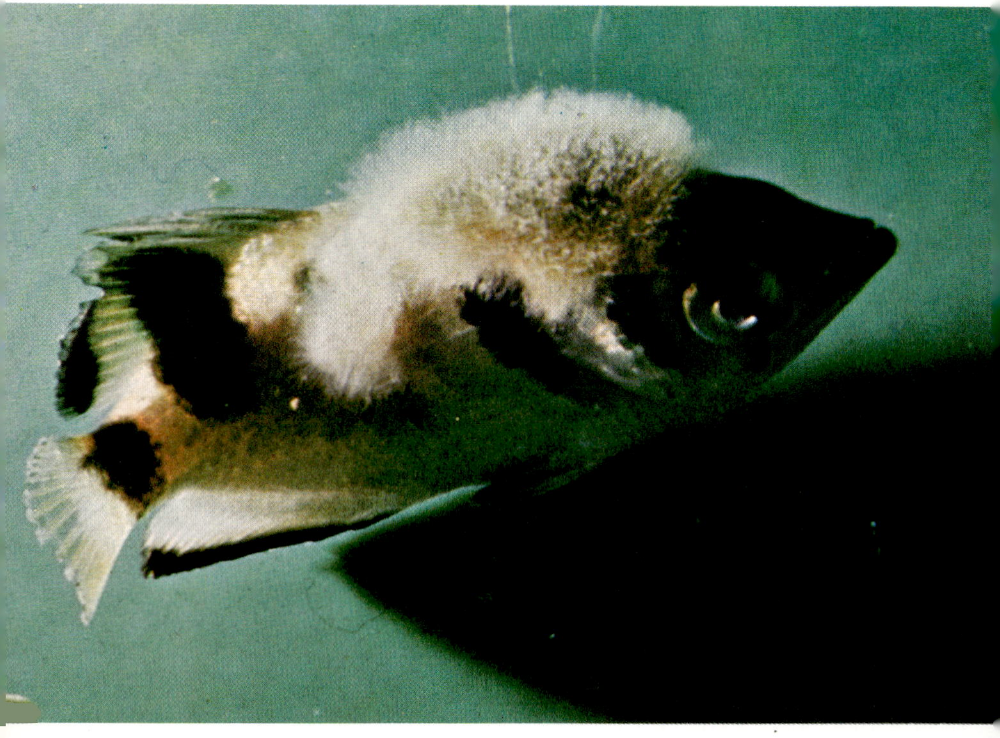

III. Parasitic Diseases

DISEASES CAUSED BY PROTOZOANS

The parasitic protozoans affecting marine aquarium fishes belong to three classes: flagellates, sporozoans and ciliates. Among these, the most common parasites are found among the flagellates. This group contains the unicellular organism *Oodinium ocellatum*, which causes velvet or coralfish disease.

Oodinium [*Amyloodinium*] *ocellatum*, the causative agent of velvet disease, is perhaps the most dreaded protozoan in the marine aquarium. These parasitic protozoans were found parasitizing the gills of *Amphiprion percula.* Photo by Frickhinger.

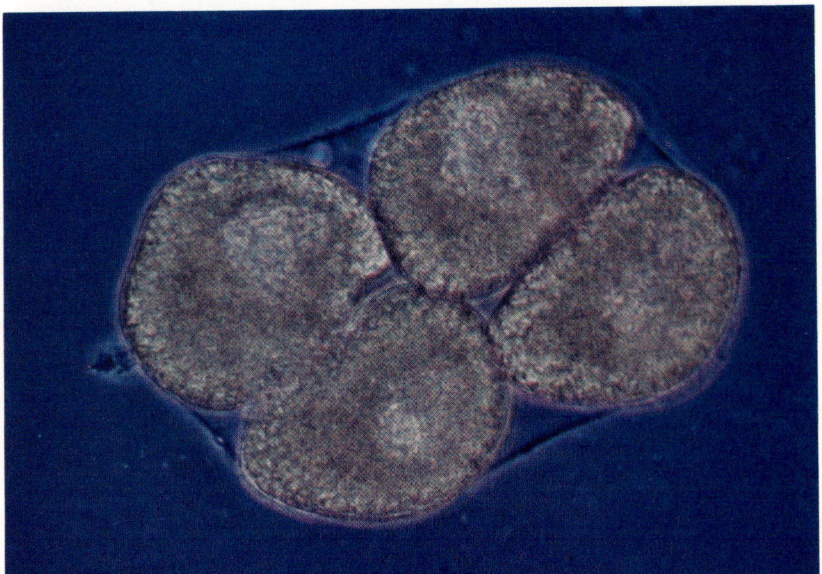

FLAGELLATES

Oodinium and Related Species

Oodinium (syn. *Amyloodinium*) *ocellatum*, a pear-shaped organism, attaches to the fishes' gills by amoeboidal roots that diverge from the parasite's body. These roots are thought to function in the uptake of nutrients as well as serving to anchor the organism to the host. Heavy accumulations of the parasites on the gill lamellae can cause the fish to suffocate.

The organism can also attack the surface of the skin, producing fine velvety lesions, hence the common name velvet disease. When examined microscopically the parasite has a single nucleus and is surrounded by a thin membrane, yellowish in color.

When the parasitic stage reaches maturation, the organism leaves the host and falls to the bottom of the tank. During this subsequent encysted stage, numerous internal divisions occur; these divisions result in the formation of many dinospores. The free-swimming dinospores then burst from the cyst in search of a host. Dinospores are green in color and have the characteristic form of a dinoflagellate. The dinospore has two flagella, one of which is in a furrow. Sometimes a red eye-spot is observed on these dinospores. Unless the dinospore successfully attached itself to a host it soon dies. The free-swimming stages are suspected of having chemotactic properties to aid them in their search for a host. Soon after attachment, the dinoflagellate loses its flagella and metamorphoses into the parasitic stage.

To assure successful treatment of velvet disease, therapy should begin in the early stages of the infection. Copper sulfate solutions, with or without other drugs, are the most widely used therapeutic agents. When copper sulfate is used alone, the recommended dosage is 0.15 ppm over a 2-week period. Successful results have also been reported by bathing affected fishes in copper

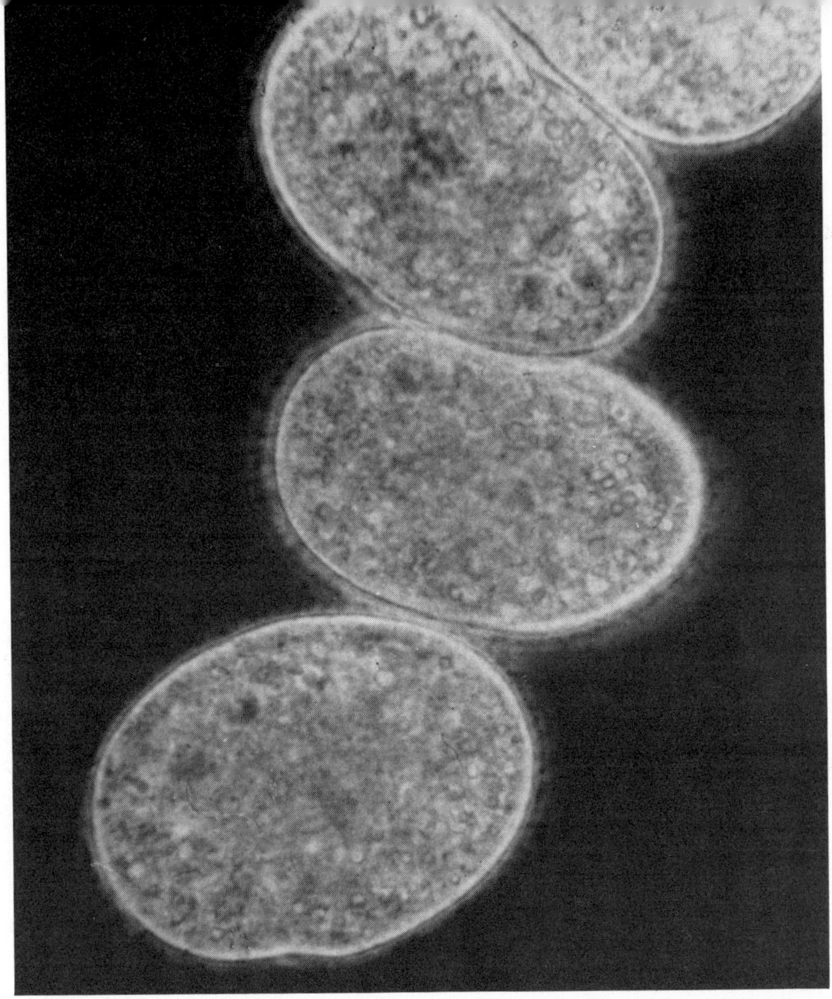

Miamiensis avidus is commonly found parasitizing the skin and gills of marine fishes. This ciliated protozoan is very similar to the freshwater ciliate *Tetrahymena.*

sulfate (0.5 mg/l) combined with Neguvon (0.5 mg/l).

Oodinium ocellatum occurs in all oceans and in brackish waters. Freshwater species include *O. limneticum* in North America and *O. pillularis* in Europe, Asia and Africa. A related dinoflagellate was found to cause severe lesions and heavy mortalities in captive marine aquarium fishes. Treatment for this pathogen, *Oodinioides vastator*, is nearly impossible. Destroying affected fishes is recommended.

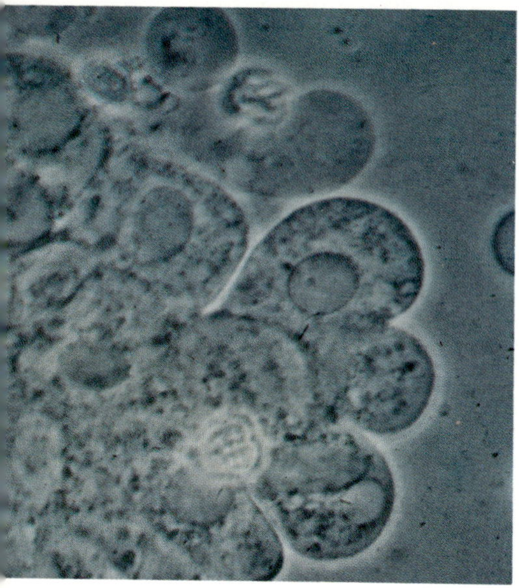

Left:
During the parasitic stage, *Oodinioides vastator* attacks the gills of marine fishes.

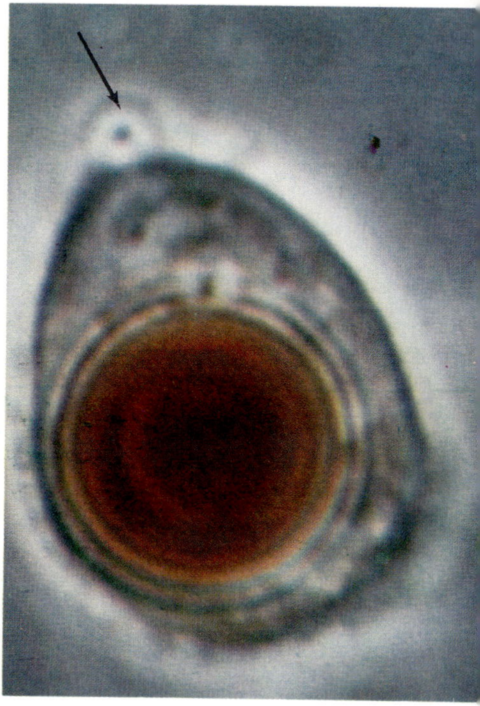

Right:
This photo depicts the beginning of sporulation in *Oodinioides vastator.* The sealed aperture (top) develops after the parasite falls from the host.

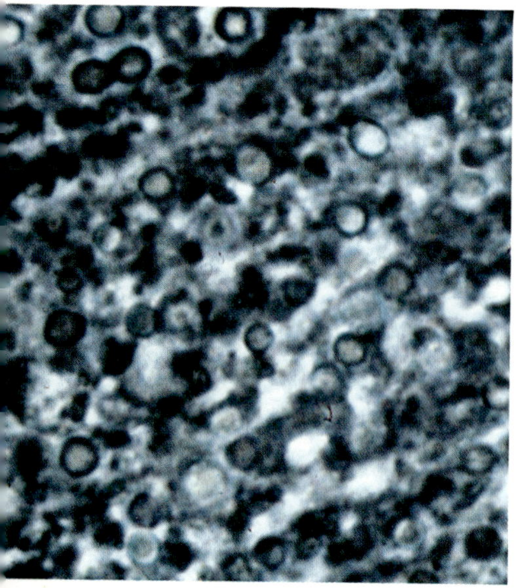

Left:
Numerous single-flagellated dinospores are released from the encysted stage to actively seek a host for attachment. Photos by Frickhinger.

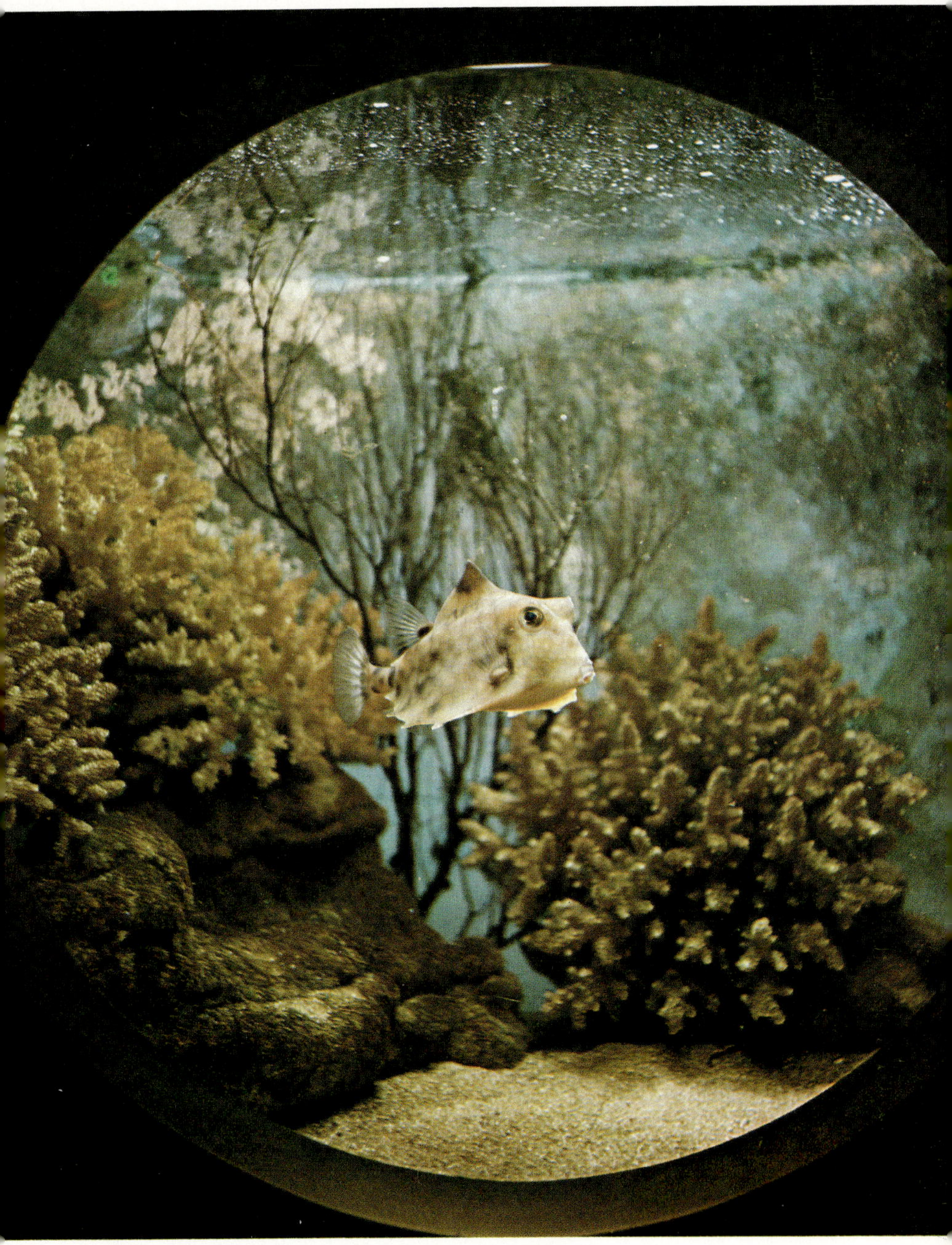

Aquarium fishes should be closely observed each day in order that behavior abnormalities and signs of disease can be promptly recognized. Photo by Dr. D. Terver, Nancy Aquarium.

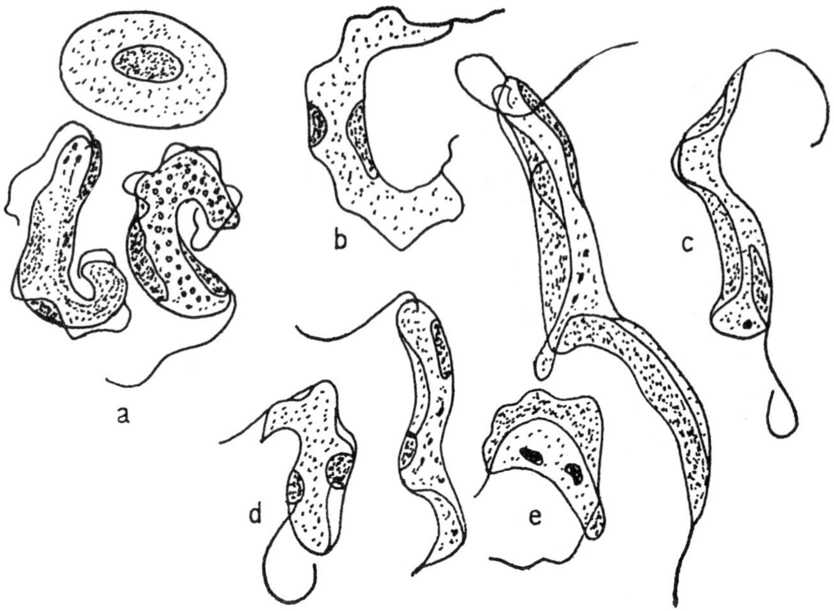

Various species of *Cryptobia* affect both marine and freshwater fishes. These blood parasites are transmitted by piscivorous leeches. Some representative species include: a. *C. acipenseris,* b. *C. barbi,* c. *C. keysselitzi,* d. *C. gurneyorum,* and e. *C. markewitschi.* After Bychowsky.

Cryptobia

Species of the genus *Cryptobia* are known to occur in the blood of various marine fishes. They are occasionally seen on blood smears, winding between the blood cells. In small numbers they do little damage; however, large numbers of *Cryptobia* cause weak-disease, a sort of "sleeping-sickness" of fishes. The disease is transmitted by piscivorous leeches. There are no reports of an effective treatment for this blood parasite.

Hexamita

Another flagellated protozoan which occurs in both fresh and salt water is *Hexamita intestinalis.* This unicellular parasite has eight flagella and normally lives in the intestine, but it is capable of penetrating the intestinal lining and entering the circulatory system. Once systemic, the parasite can penetrate the subcutis and emerge, thereby causing tubular eruptions. Successful treatment involves the use of either the Italian drug emtrysidine or the American product Flagyl®

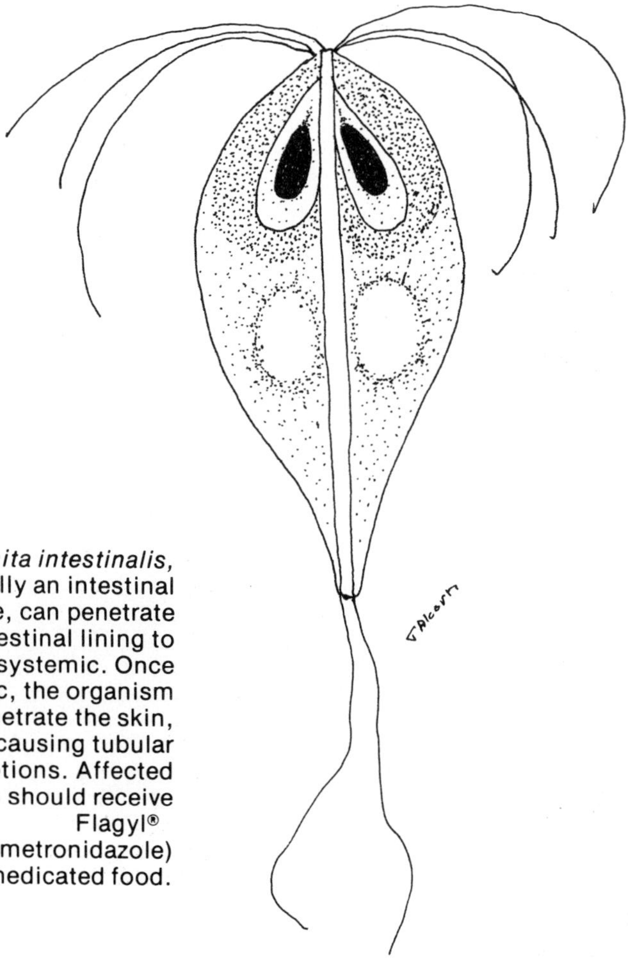

Hexamita intestinalis, initially an intestinal parasite, can penetrate the intestinal lining to become systemic. Once systemic, the organism can penetrate the skin, causing tubular eruptions. Affected fishes should receive Flagyl® (metronidazole) medicated food.

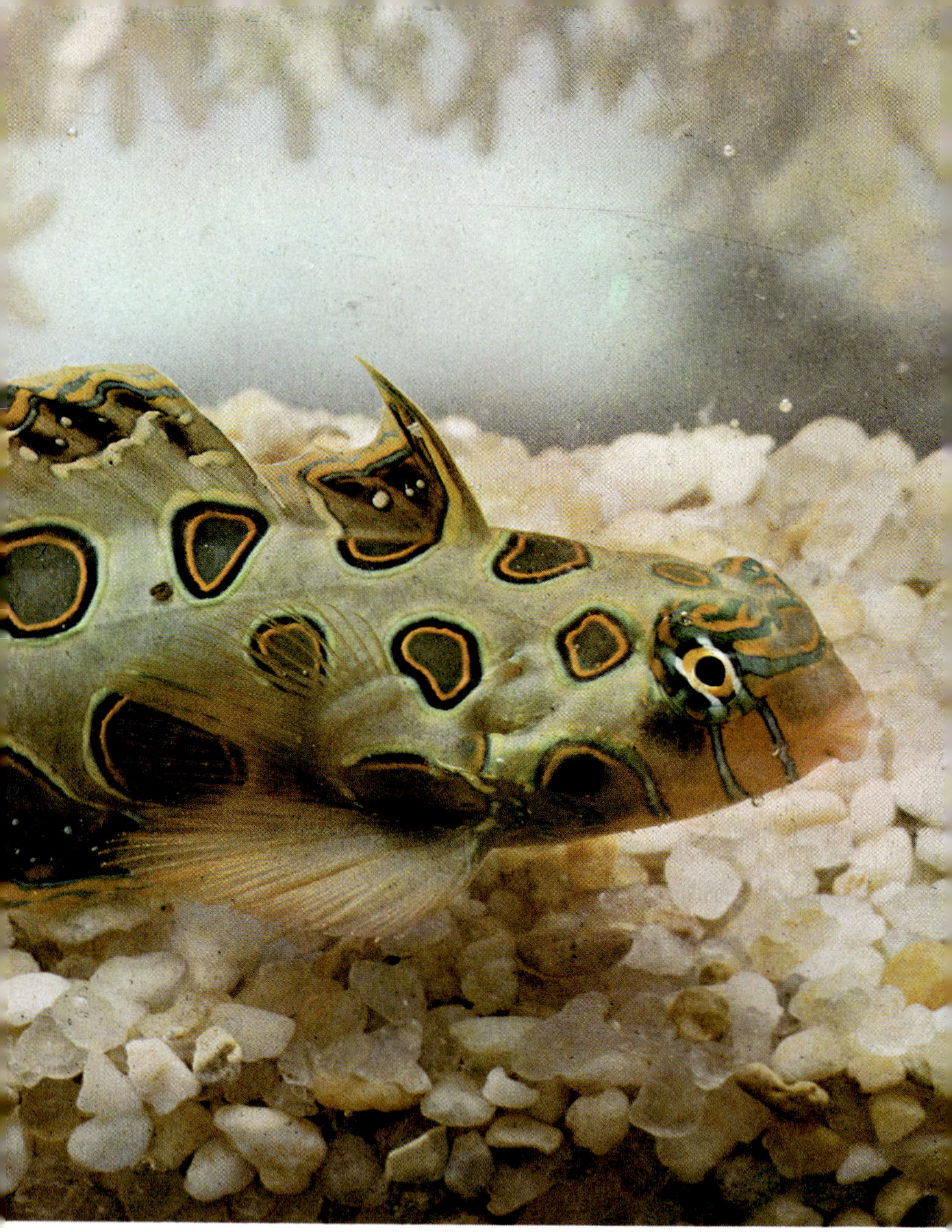

The aquarist should become thoroughly familiar with the normal coloration of his captive fishes. This spectacularly colored dragonet, *Synchiropus splendida,* exhibits normal coloration. A progressive loss of color is suggestive of a chronic bacterial disease such as tuberculosis. Photo by Dr. Herbert R. Axelrod.

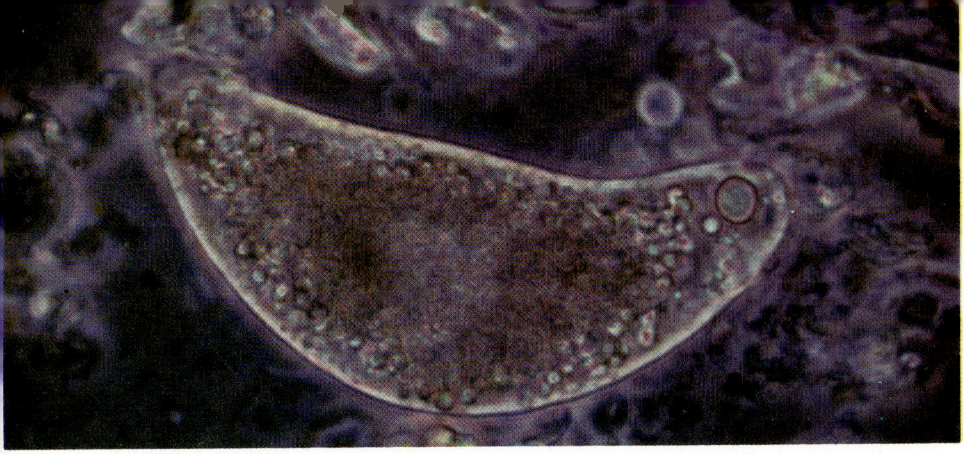

Balantidium sp. is an intestinal parasite of marine fishes. This ciliated protozoan was found in the large intestine of *Heniochus acuminatus.* Photo by Frickhinger.

There are over 200 species of venomous marine fishes. Perhaps the most dangerous and undoubtedly the ugliest group of venomous piscines are the stonefishes. Because a stonefish is often adorned with other benthic dwellers such as algae, its remarkable camouflage makes it practically undetectable. The sting of this species, *Synanceia verrucosa,* may be lethal unless specific anti-venom is administered. Photo by Dr. Shih-chieh Shen.

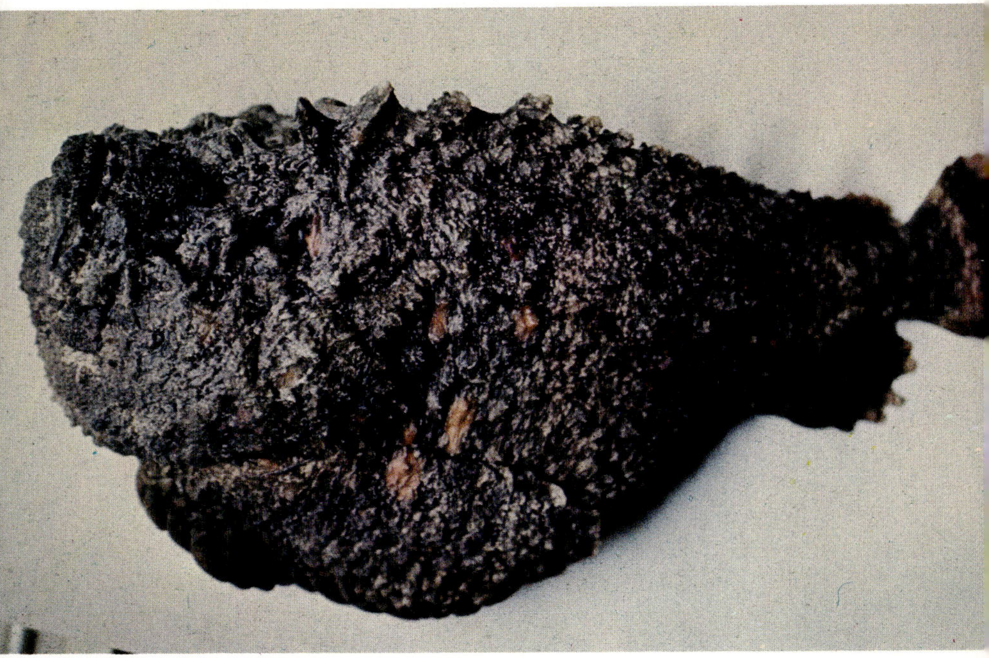

SPOROZOANS

Sporozoan parasites also represent a severe threat to the health of marine aquarium fishes. These protozoans can invade the gills, subcutis, muscles, blood and various internal organs. In some cases they cause little harm, whereas at other times they are responsible for extensive damage.

Coccidia

Eimeria and *Hemogregarina* (class Sporozoa, order Coccidia) are two parasitic genera of marine fishes. *Eimeria* sp. have been found in the testes and liver of clupeoid fishes. Hemogregarines are intracellular blood parasites and are transmitted by an invertebrate host. Recently, sporozoans were found in hypertrophied monocytes in the blood of cultured turbots (*Scophthalmus maximus*) (14). These parasites were reported to be *Toxoplasma*-like in appearance (21).

Eimeria sardinae spores. After Kabata.

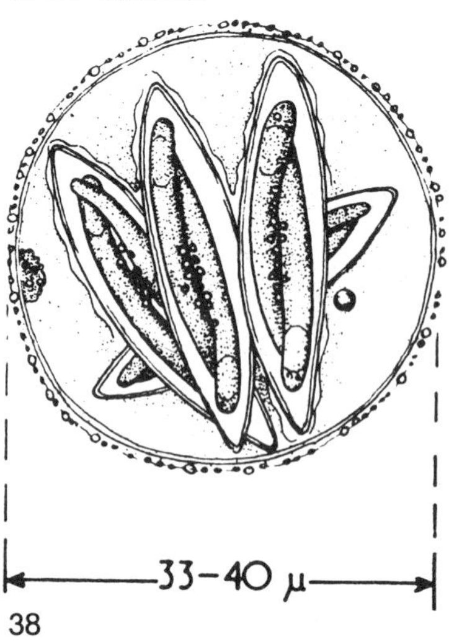

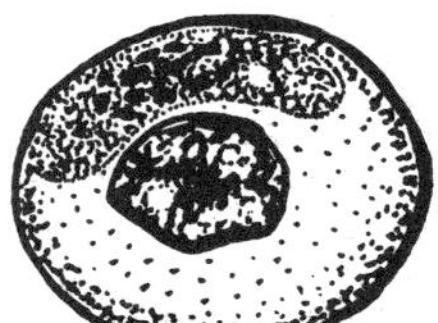

Hemogregarina bigemina within an erythrocyte. After Laird.

Hemogregarina irkadukisiki within an erythrocyte. After Laird.

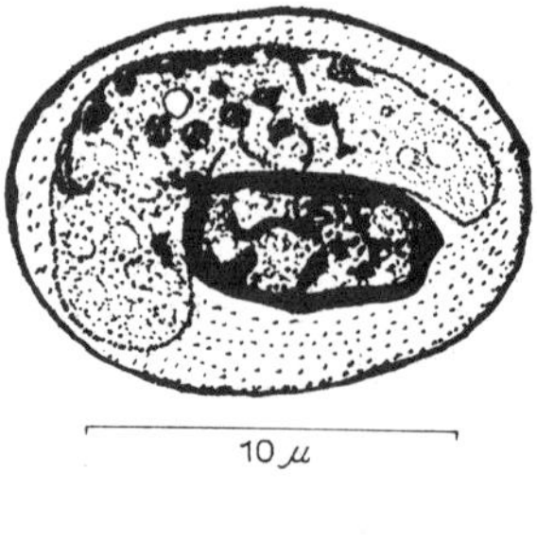

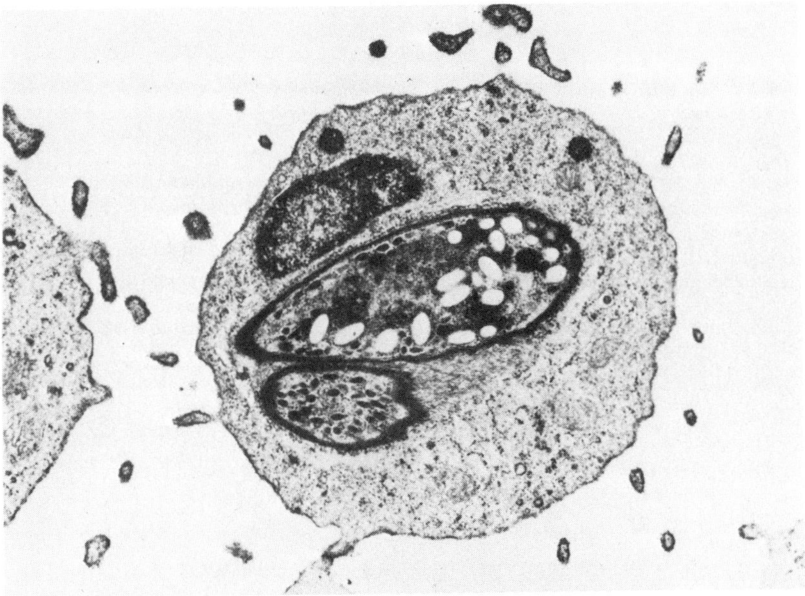

This electron photomicrograph reveals two trophozoites within a hypertrophied monocyte. These parasitic sporozoans closely resemble *Toxoplasma.* Photo by Ferguson and Roberts.

Myxosporidia

Myxosporidian parasites have been reported in a variety of marine fishes. These organisms are classified according to rather distinctive morphological features of the spores. The polar capsules and the filaments they contain are among the most unique morphological features of the myxosporidian spore. Myxosporidia spores have two polar capsules; microsporidia have only one. When the parasite is touching the host substrate, the so-called cnidocil at the top of the spore opens the capsule and a long filament is extruded. This filament is thought to have an anchoring function while the plasmodium is freed to penetrate the host's tissue. The plasmodial stages, or trophozoites, have a very limited use in taxonomy, making it nearly impossible to determine the particular species when only trophozoites are found.

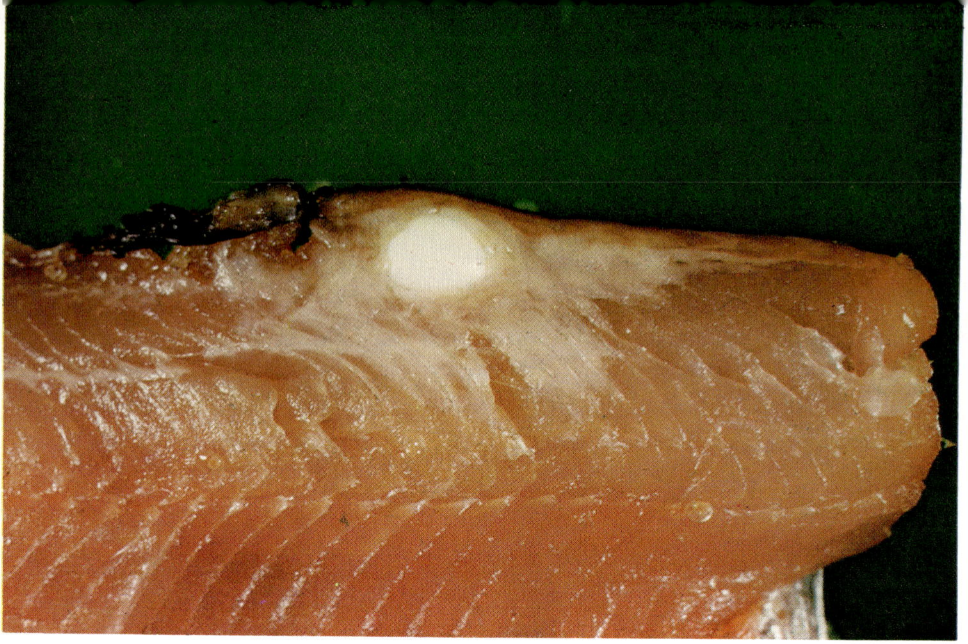

Histozoic myxosporidia of the genus *Henneguya* were responsible for causing this cystic lesion; these cysts are filled with developing or mature spores. A microscopic view of the *Henneguya* spore (below) reveals the characteristic double caudal processes which help identify this genus. Photos by Frickhinger.

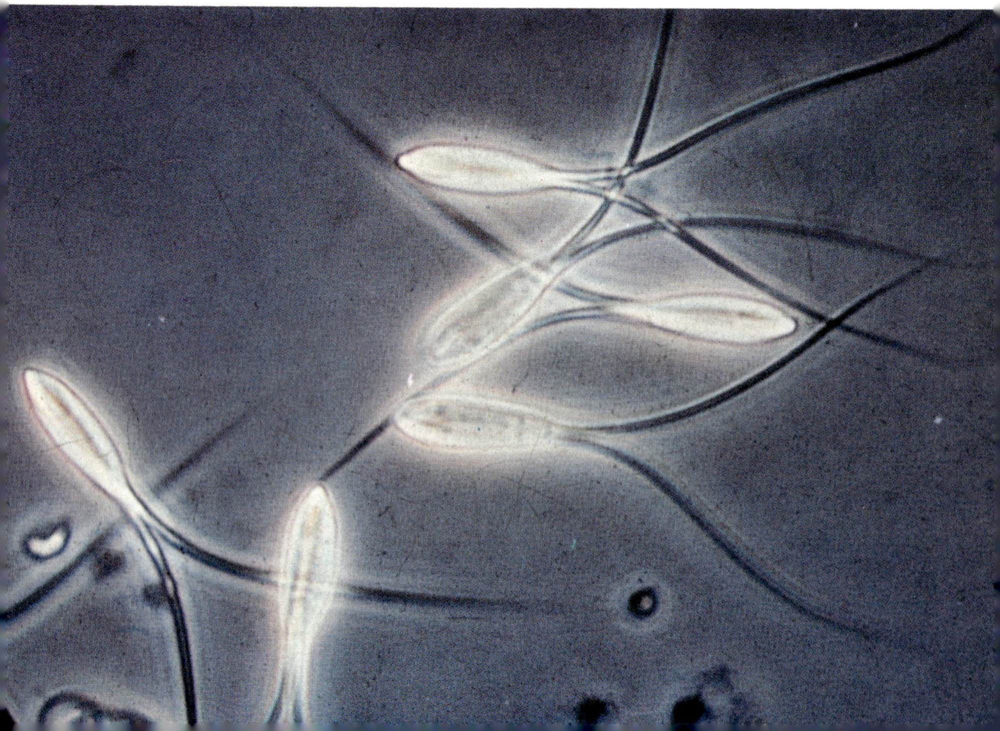

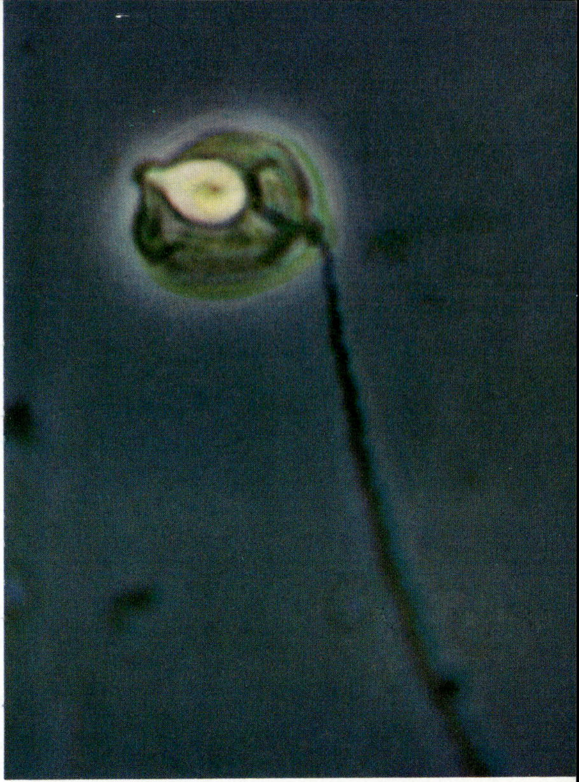

Myxosporidians are commonly found parasitizing the gall bladder of various marine fishes. Both *Ceratomyxa* sp. (right with polar filament extruded) and *Myxidium* sp. (below) were recovered from the gall bladder of *Cyclichthys antennatus.* Photos by Frickhinger.

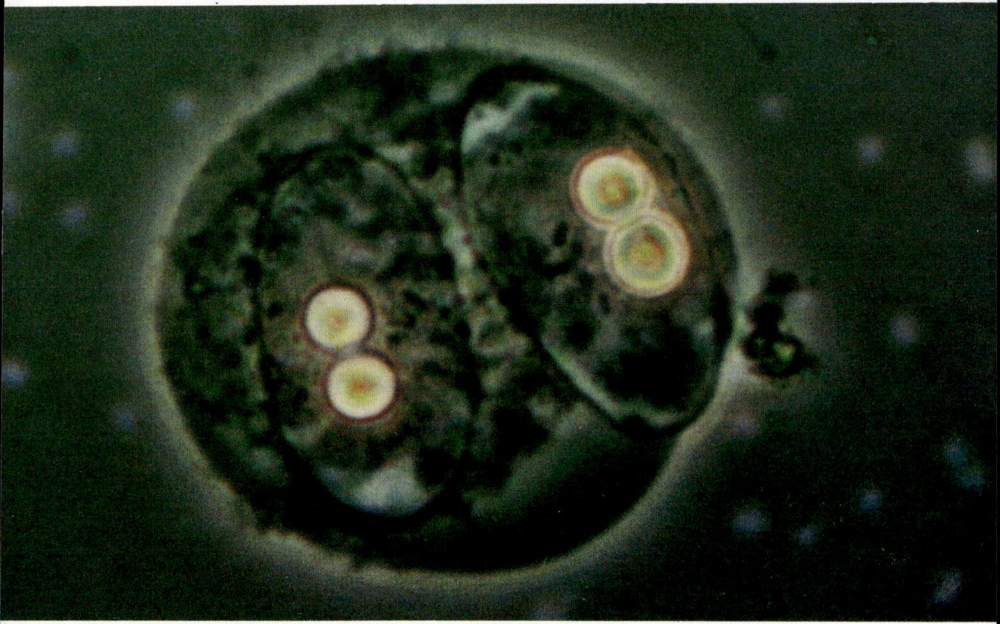

At a later stage in the infection the trophozoites have grown and the nucleus multiplies to a syncytium. In this syncytium the characteristic spores finally are developed; they can be identified on the basis of morphological characteristics. Some of the most common myxosporidia which have been distinguished on the basis of spore morphology include the genera *Myxobolus*, *Myxidium*, *Henneguya*, *Chloromyxum*, *Kudoa* and *Ceratomyxa*.

A variety of spore shapes exist among the myxosporidia; some representative examples include: 16. *Myxobolus aeglefini*, 17. *Myxidium gadi*, 18. *Ceratomyxa macrospora*, 19. *Ceratomyxa drepanopsettae*, 20. *Sphaeromyxa balbianii* and 21. *Auerbachia* sp. Photos by Dr. Jiri Lom.

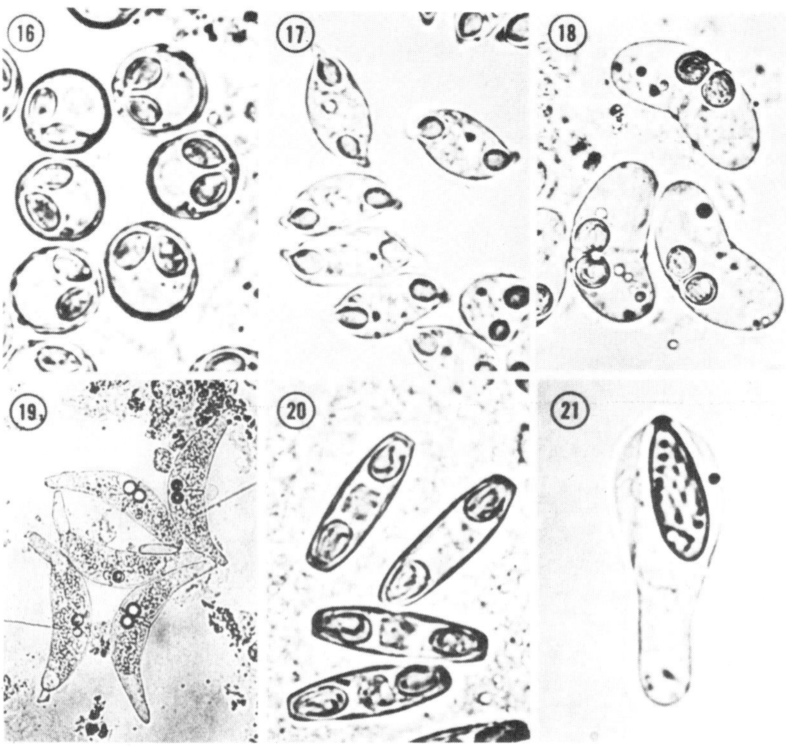

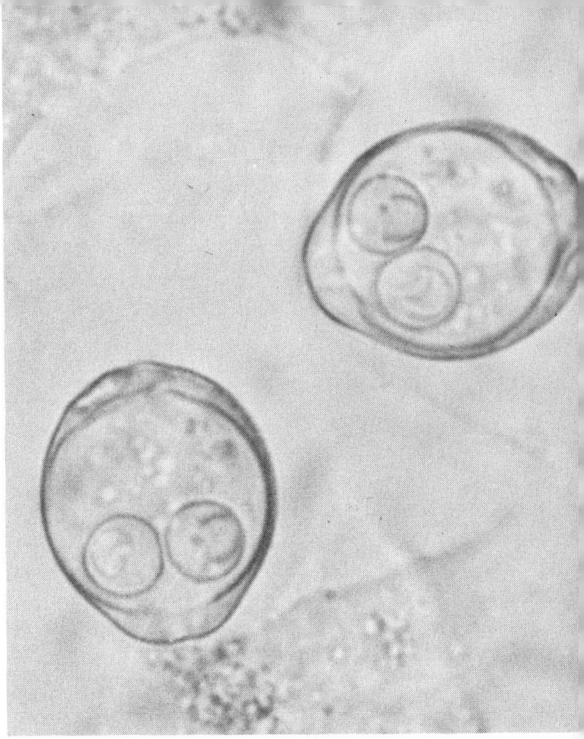

Most myxosporidia of marine fishes are found in the gall bladder or urinary bladder. These myxospores were recovered from the kidney of *Mugil auratus*. Photo by Arnal, San Pedro del Pinatar, Murcia, Spain.

Myxobolus spores are pear-shaped. These parasites often become localized in the gills where they become enclosed in little white cysts. Generally they cause only minor pathological changes. There is no known treatment. Species of *Myxidium* have been observed in the blood and tissues of eels. Species of *Chloromyxum* and *Kudoa* become localized in the musculature and are responsible for causing a "milky" or grayish discoloration of the muscle. Sometimes cysts occur beneath the skin or on the fins and body. These cysts contain spores which are elongate or cuboidal in shape. *Henneguya* spores also can become localized in different tissues. Their sporocysts often become visible as white nodules under the skin and on the gills and fins. Diagnosis is made based upon identification of typical spores with two "tails." Another myxosporidian, *Unicapsula muscularis*, was reported to cause muscle infections in *Maena smaris* in the Mediterranean (59).

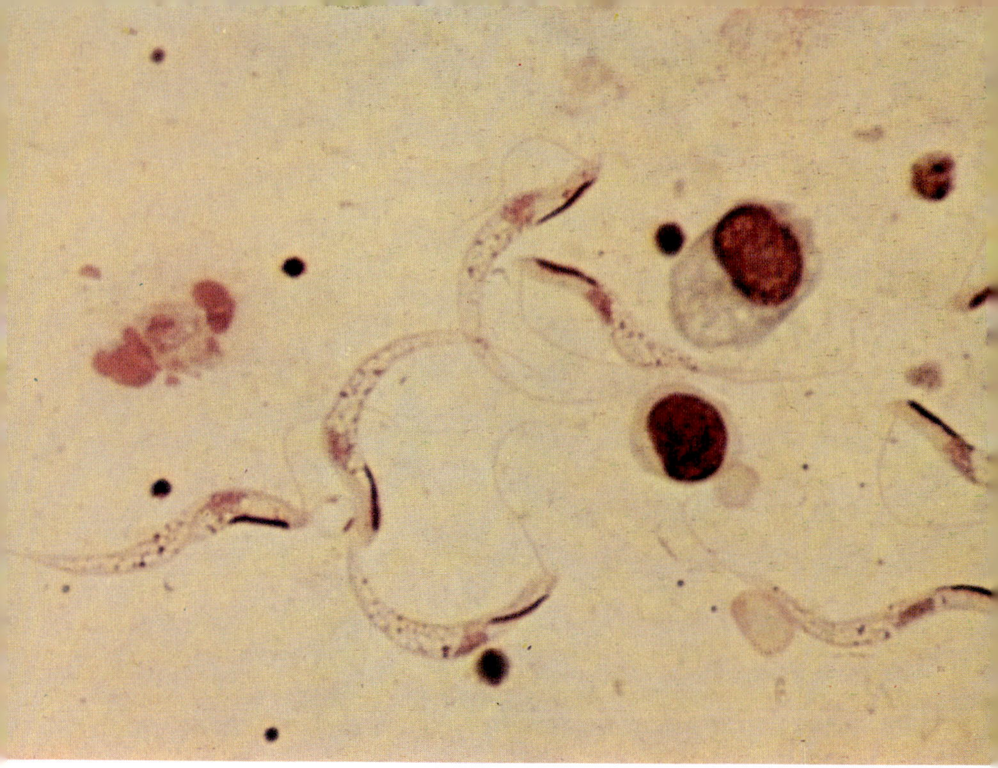

This stained blood smear reveals numerous *Cryptobia* sp. These hemoflagellates can also be detected on unstained smears as they meander about the blood cells. Photo by Dr. Becker.

Parasitic helminths have been found in almost all fish tissues. These microfilaria were found within the eye of *Tetraodon palembangensis.* Photo by Frickhinger.

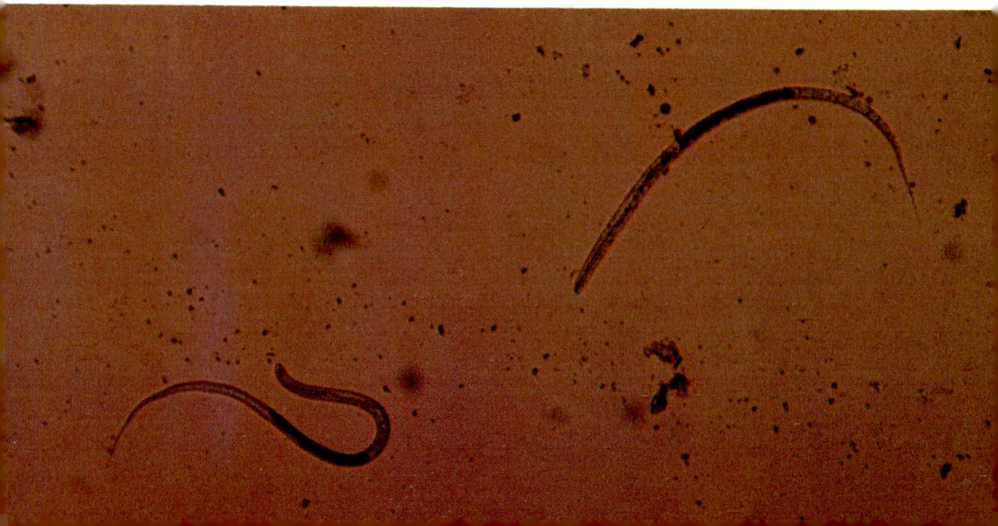

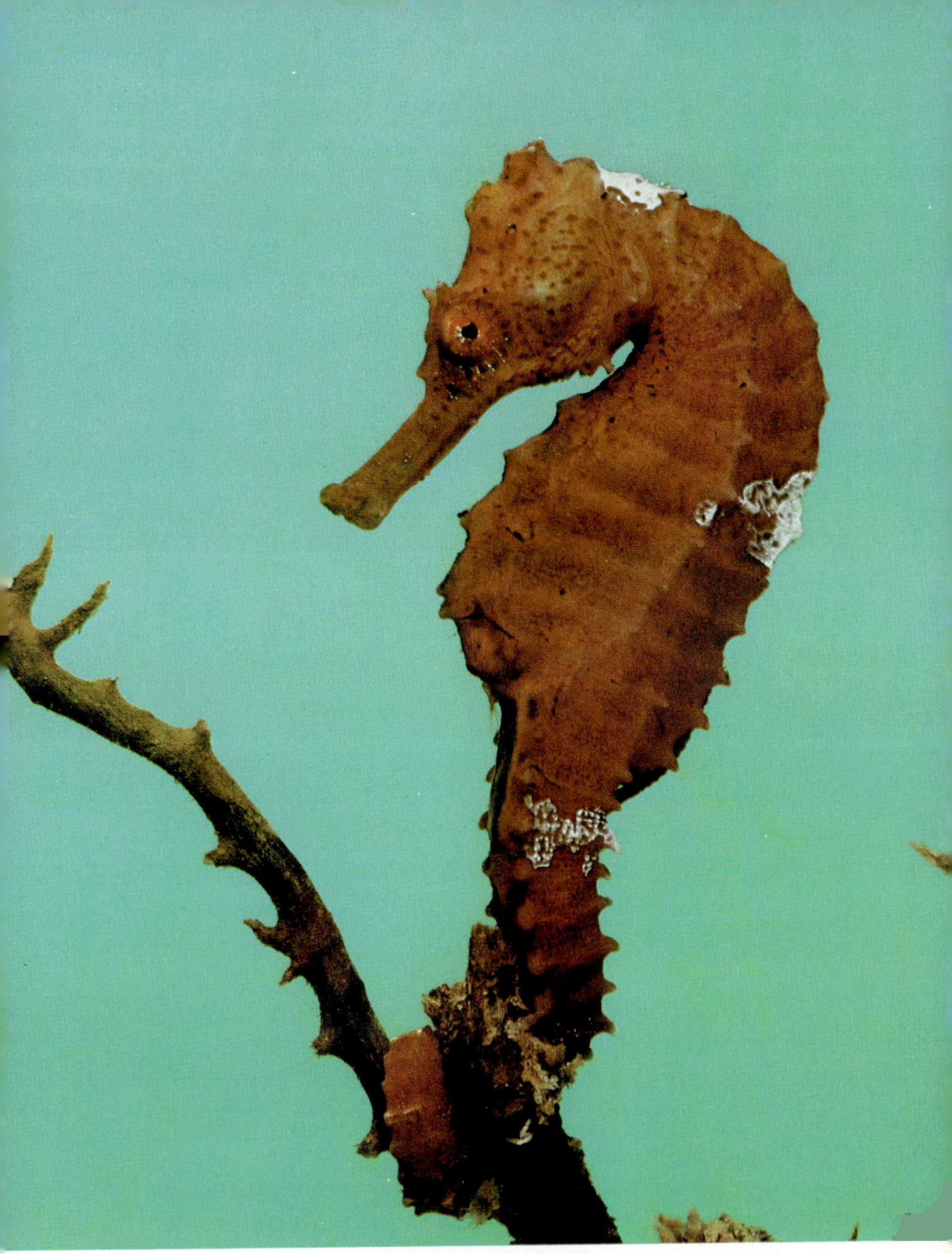

When seahorses become infected with microsporidia, loss of color generally precedes the appearance of skin lesions. *Glugea* and *Plistophora* sp. are commonly recovered from cystic muscular lesions such as those shown on this seahorse. Photo by Marine Studios, Marineland, Florida.

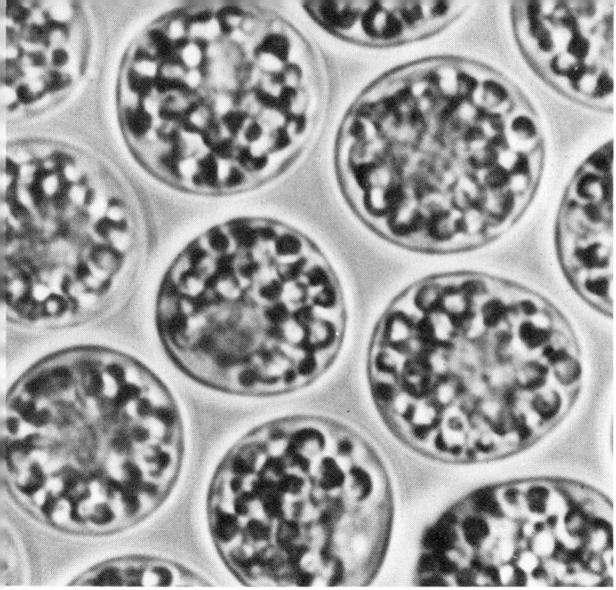

This high-powered (X 5000) photomicrograph reveals numerous *Dermocystidium* spores within a single gill cyst. Photo by Dr. Jiri Lom.

Microsporidia and Haplosporidia

Another order in the class Sporozoa is Microsporidia. As mentioned earlier, Microsporidia have only one polar capsule. These parasites are frequently reported to infect marine fishes; generally they occur in the musculature and liver. Members of the genus *Glugea* are responsible for heavy infections of marine fishes. *Glugea* sp. cause varying degrees of visceral involvement and can lead to the death of the host.

Infections with the microsporidian *Nosema* have resulted in the formation of large tumor-like cysts in the central nervous system. Several species of *Plistophora* have caused intramuscular cysts of marine fishes. When a seahorse becomes infected with this parasite the muscles become pale and the fish's body becomes discolored.

Infections with *Dermocystidium* (Haplosporidia) cause whitish round to elongate cysts in the subcutis, gills and musculature of marine fishes. These cysts contain masses of rounded, operculated spores. There is no known treatment for any of the myxosporidians, microsporidians or *Dermocystidium*.

CILIATES

Cryptocaryon irritans is the most common and widely known ciliated protozoan capable of causing disease in marine aquarium fishes. It is closely related to *Ichthyophthirius*, the ciliated protozoan which causes "ich" of freshwater fishes. *Cryptocaryon* is an external parasite of the gills and skin. Oftentimes the parasite penetrates the epidermis, making successful treatment rather difficult.

Because numerous white spots appear on the skin and fins of fishes affected with *Cryptocaryon,* the name white spot disease is commonly applied to this type of involvement. If untreated, death can occur within 3 to 5 days after the appearance of these papules. Photo by Herkner.

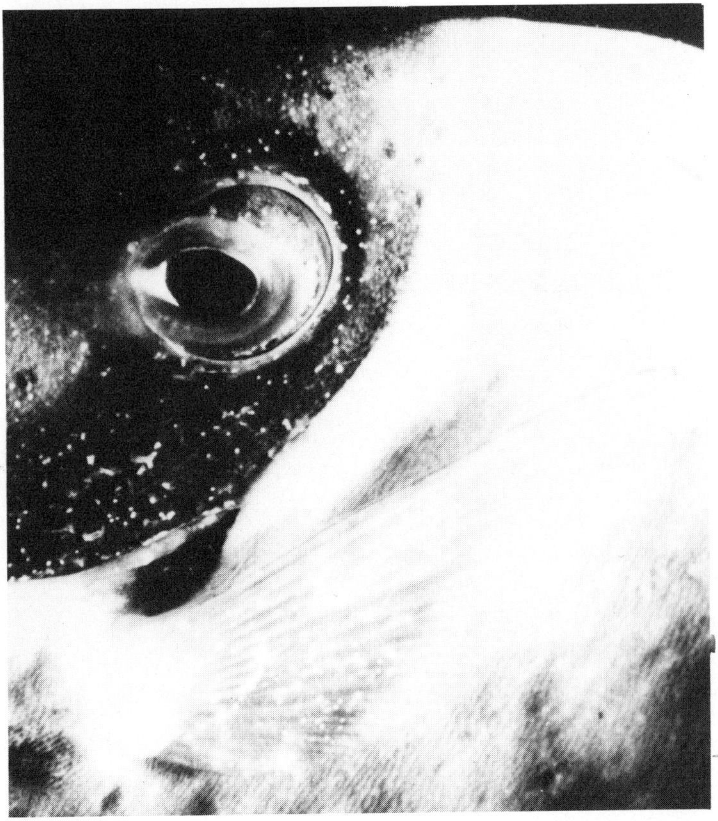

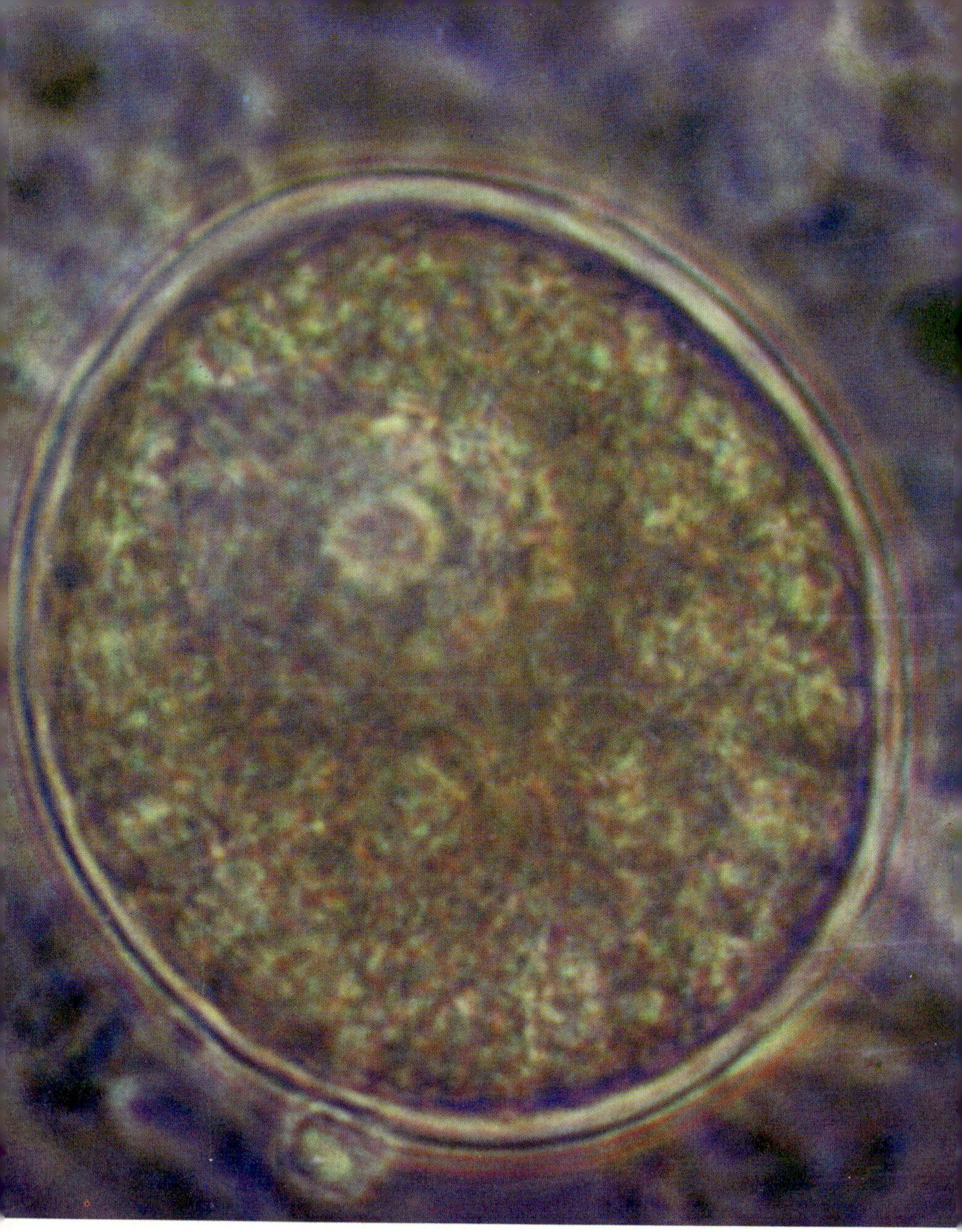

The parasitic form of *Cryptocaryon irritans* is oval to round and holotrichously ciliated; it typically has a U-shaped macronucleus and a small micronucleus. Like *Ichthyophthirius*, it falls from the host when mature and develops an encysted stage. Multiple divisions result in the formation of hundreds of swarmers which are released in search of a host. Photo by Frickhinger.

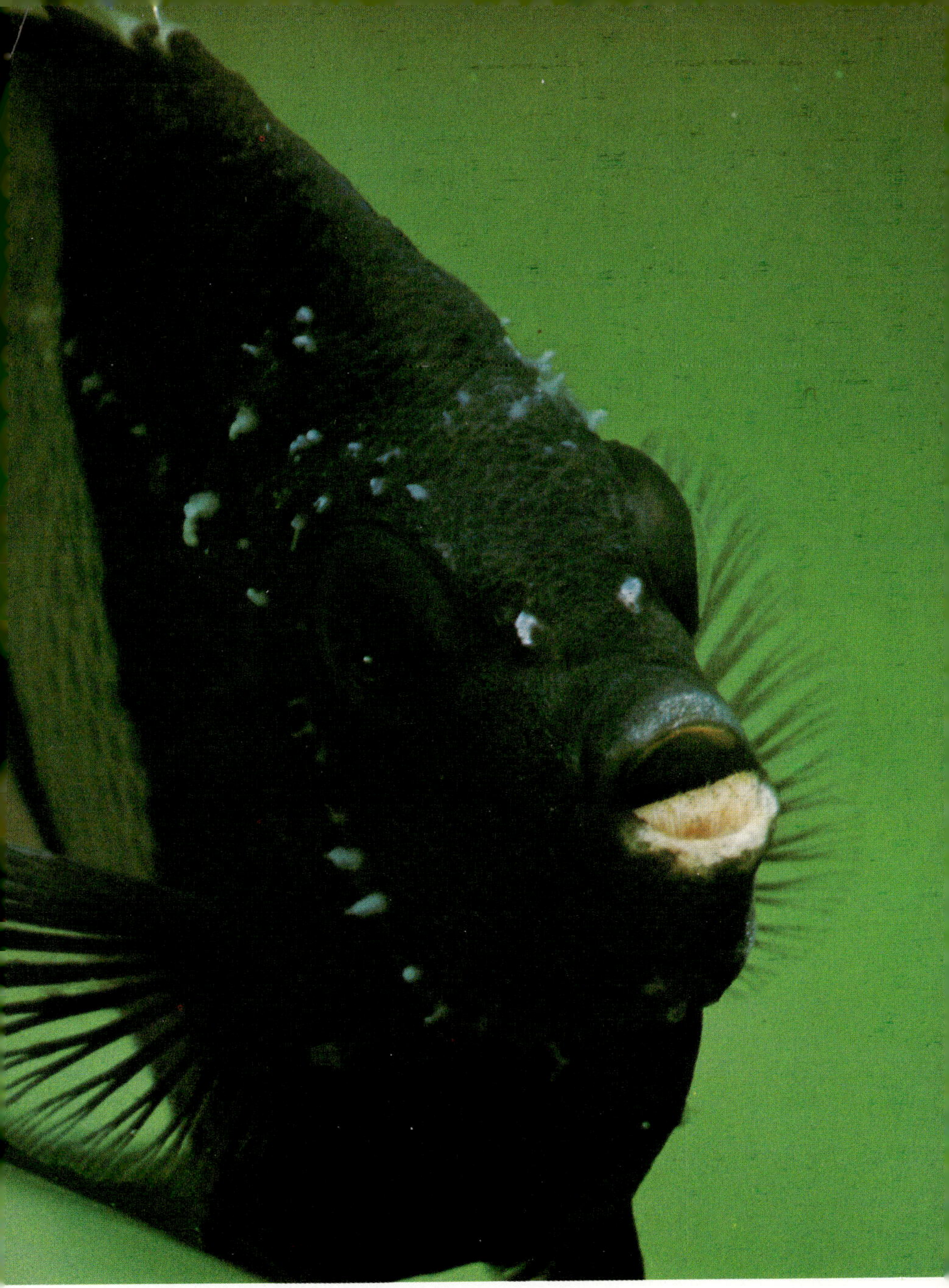

This *Arusetta asfur* is suffering from a heavy *Cryptocaryon* infection. Long-duration copper sulfate baths are commonly used to control this parasite. Photo by Frickhinger.

The adult parasite is round to oval in shape and holotrichously ciliated; it typically has a U-shaped macronucleus and a small micronucleus. Like *Ichthyophthirius*, it falls from the host when mature and develops an encysted stage. Multiple divisions result in the formation of hundreds of swarmers which are released in search of a host.

Therapeutic agents are not reported to effectively destroy the developing swarmers in the encysted stage; however, various chemicals are successfully employed to kill free swimming and parasitic stages. Copper sulfate (0.15 ppm) is often used over a two week period. Another treatment involves the use of a Tris buffer, cupric acetate and formalin mixture (36). In other cases a solution of 0.15 to 0.2 mg of copper-sulfate-citric acid combined with a 1% methylene blue solution was successful. Another bath involved the use of Neguvon (0.5

One of the less common genera of parasitic ciliates is *Balantidium*. This organism was found attacking the gill tissues of a marine fish. Photo by Frickhinger.

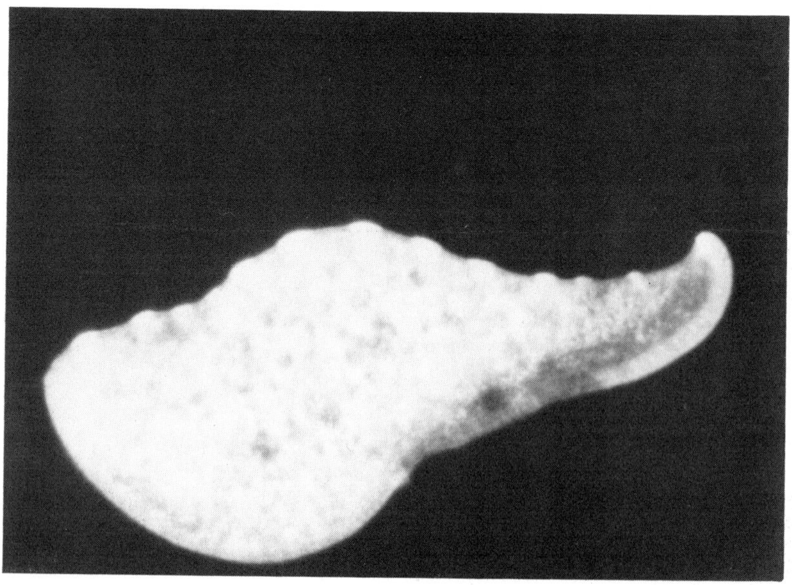

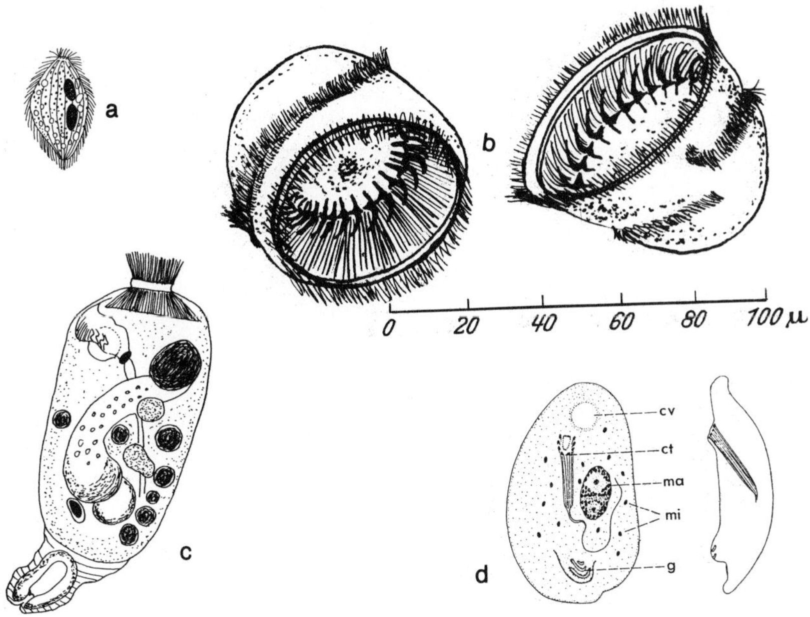

Some of the less common ciliated protozoans of marine fishes include: a. *Hemiophrys*, b. *Trichodina*, c. *Caliperia* and d. *Brooklynella hostilis*. This ventral view of *Brooklynella* reveals the contractile vacuole (cv.), cytopharyngeal tube (ct.), macronucleus (ma.), micronuclei (mi.) and glandular adhesive organelle (g.). After Lom.

mg/l) combined with copper sulfate (0.5 mg/l) (66). The free swimming and parasitic stages can also be killed by using a long-term bath in acriflavine (neutral trypaflavine) at the rate of 1 g/100 l. This should be repeated in 20 days to destroy those parasites which may have been formerly protected during the encysted stage of development.

Compared to the incidence of *Cryptocaryon*, other ciliated protozoan parasites are relatively rare in the marine environment. *Brooklynella*, a parasite closely related to the freshwater genus *Chilodonella*, has been observed attacking the gills of marine fishes. All external infections with ciliated protozoans can be eliminated by the same methods listed for treating the free swimming stages of *Cryptocaryon*.

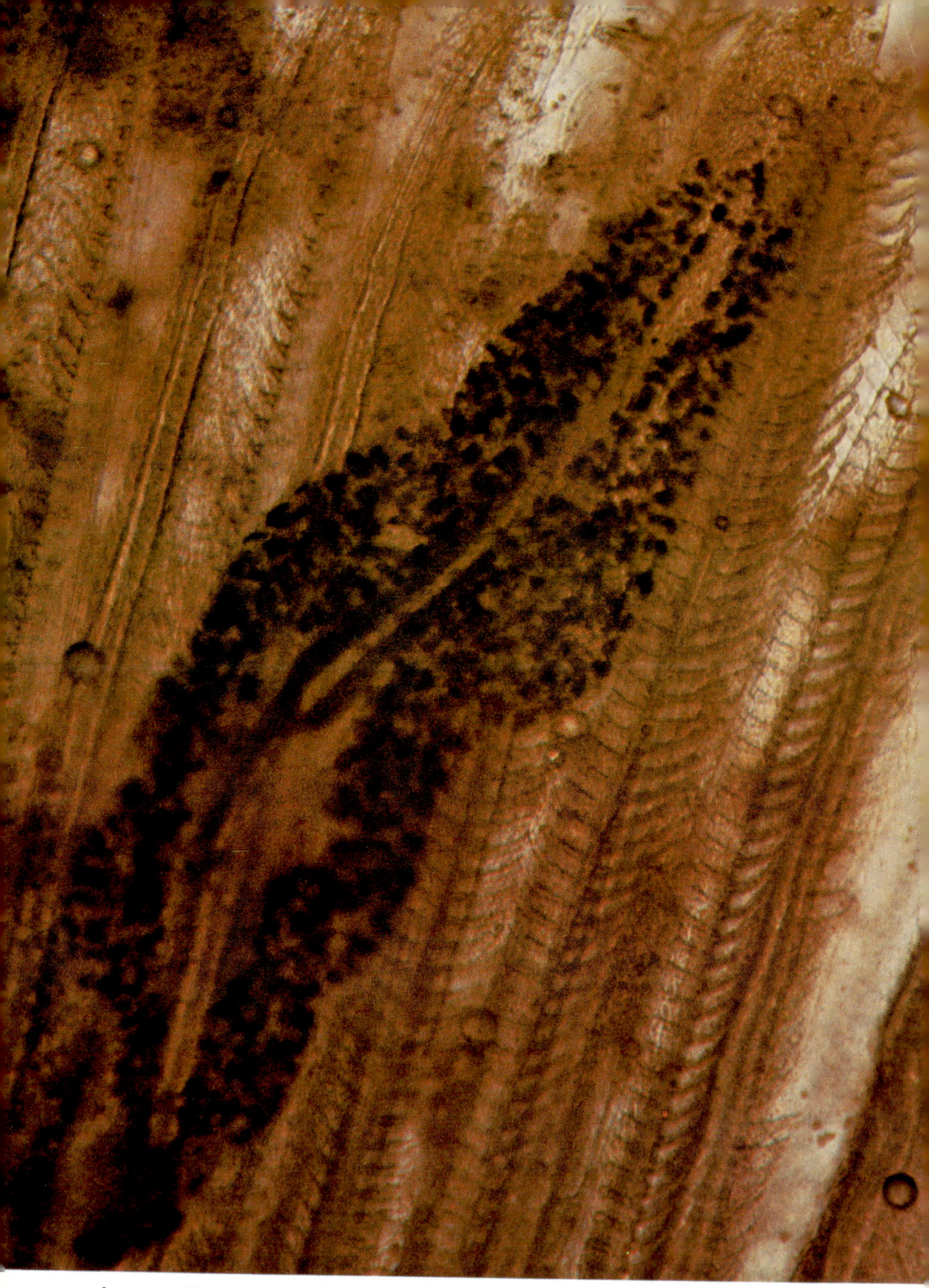

Among the monogenetic trematodes, *Microcotyle* sp. are most commonly found parasitizing the gills of marine fishes. It is easy to see how heavy infestations could severely impair respiration. Photo by Frickhinger.

DISEASES CAUSED BY HELMINTHS

Parasitic helminths have been observed on the gills and skin of marine fishes as well as in the intestine, within body organs and beneath the skin. In many cases intermediate hosts are involved in the life cycle and transmission of parasitic helminths. In these instances the helminths present the greatest problem in newly imported fishes.

Parasitic nematodes such as this species of *Contracaecum* are often found within a marine fish's intestinal tract. A variety of anthelmintics have been successfully used to remove intestinal roundworms. Photo by Frickhinger.

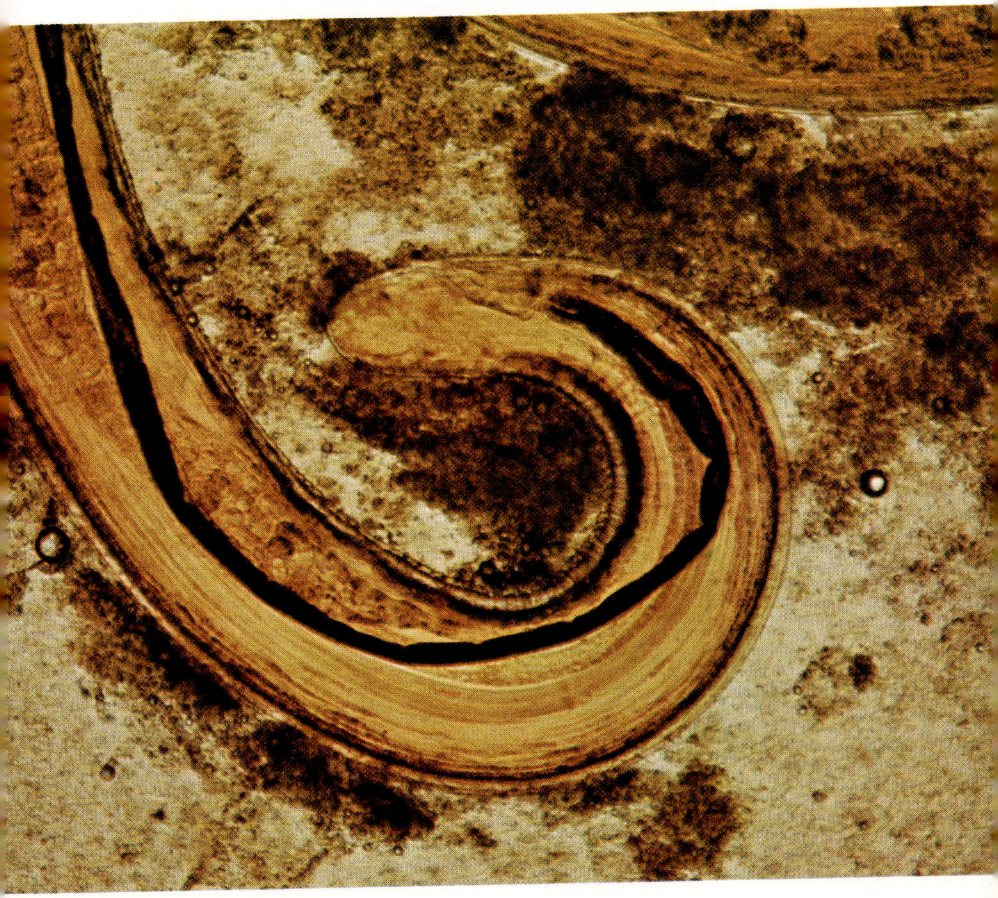

TREMATODES (FLUKES)

Monogenetic Trematodes

Monogenetic trematodes are parasitic helminths that do not require an intermediate host. Their development occurs directly on the host or in the aquarium via the development of free swimming larval forms which emerge to either reinfect the original host or infect a new host. These worms rarely cause problems in the natural environment; however, the marine aquarium provides optimum conditions for reinfestation. There are 145 species of monogeneans, the genus *Microcotyle*

Microcotyle centropristis. a. adult fluke, b. genital aperture, cirrus, c. fixation hooks and d. egg. After Reichenbach-Klinke.

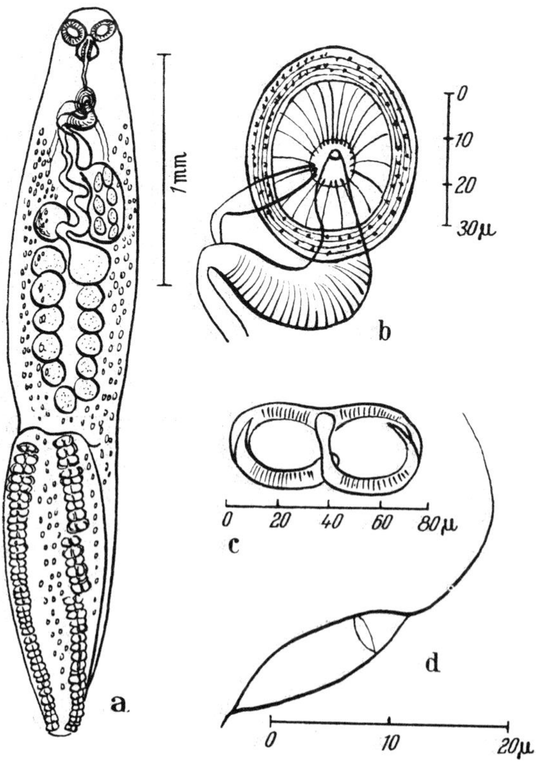

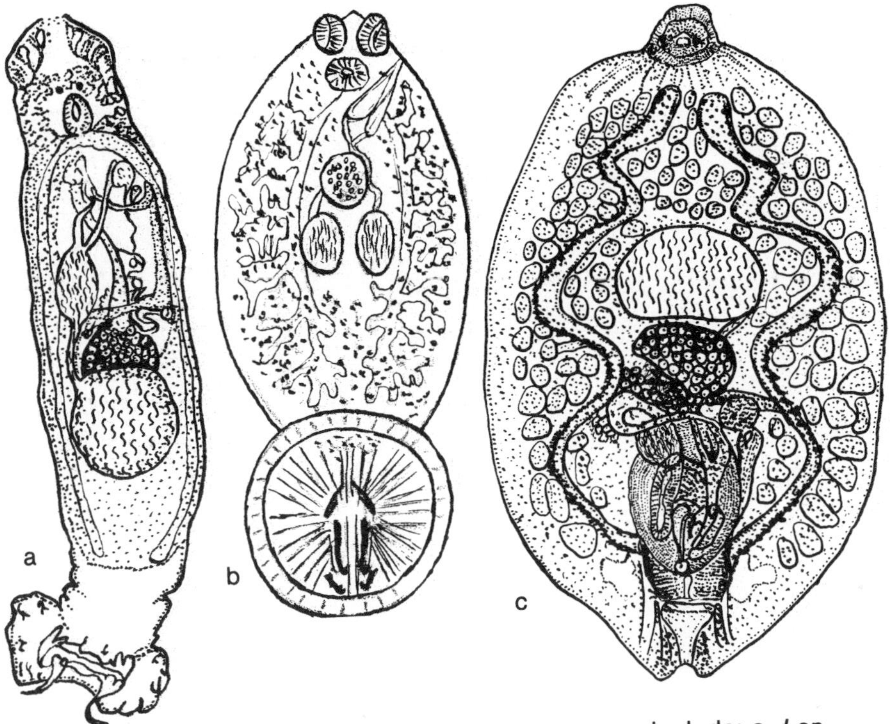

Other examples of monogeneans include: a. *Leptocotyle minor* (after Sproston), a frequent gill parasite of Mediterranean sharks, b. *Benedenia monticelli* (after Palombi) and c. *Ancyrocephalus bassensis* (after Murray).

being the most common. In one year the New York Aquarium reported that 44 fishes were infected by *Microcotyle* (35). These elongate flukes have numerous hooks on the body so they can attach themselves to the gills of marine fishes. Heavy infestations can severely impair respiratory functions.

Successful treatments for the removal of monogenetic flukes include short formalin baths (100 ml/100 l); long-term baths in acriflavine (1 g/100 l); baths in quinine sulfate or quinine hydrochloride (1 g/50 l); or baths in 0.2% potassium permanganate.

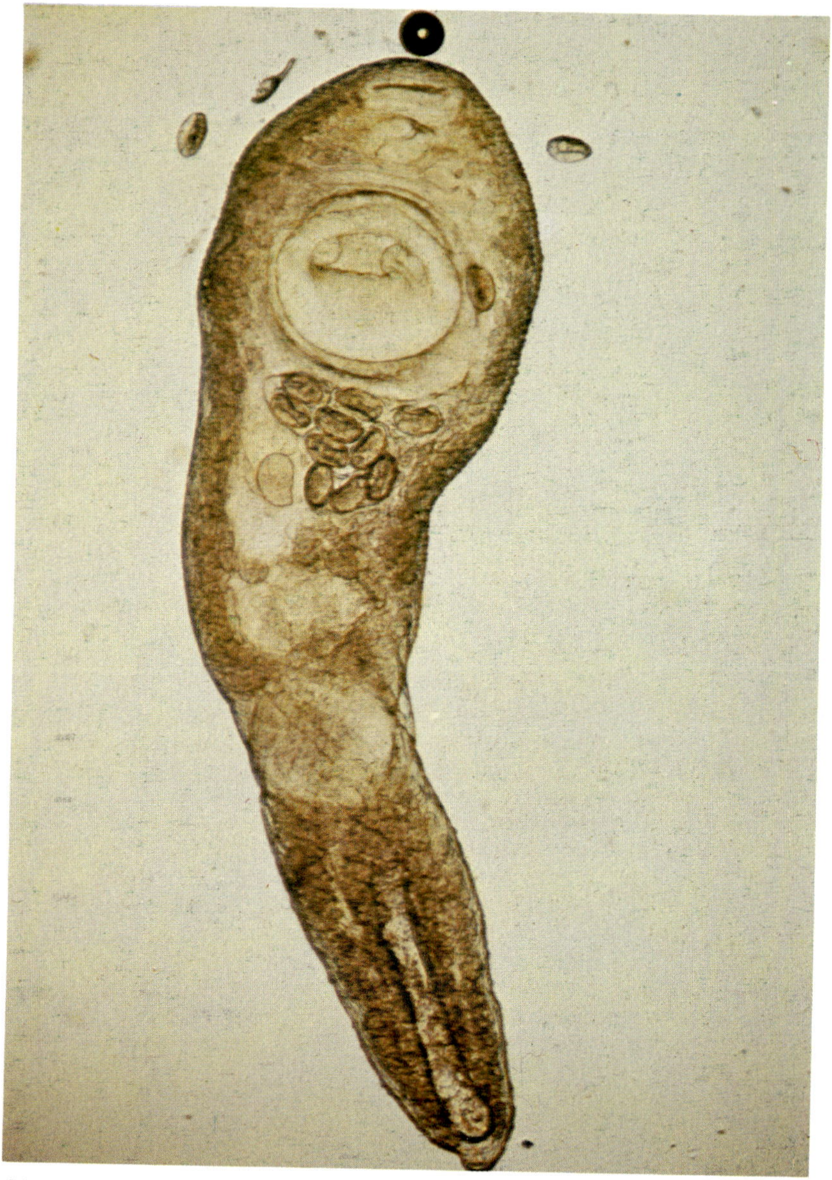

Above and opposite: Digenetic flukes such as this are not uncommonly found within newly captured marine fishes. The larval stages (opposite, above) are often found within various abdominal organs. Piscivorous birds such as the seagull (opposite, below) are often involved in the life cycle of these flukes, as are molluscs. Because of the involved life cycle of the Digenea, these flukes are not apt to be a chronic problem in the marine aquarium. Fluke photos by Frickhinger. Seagull photo by K. Gillett.

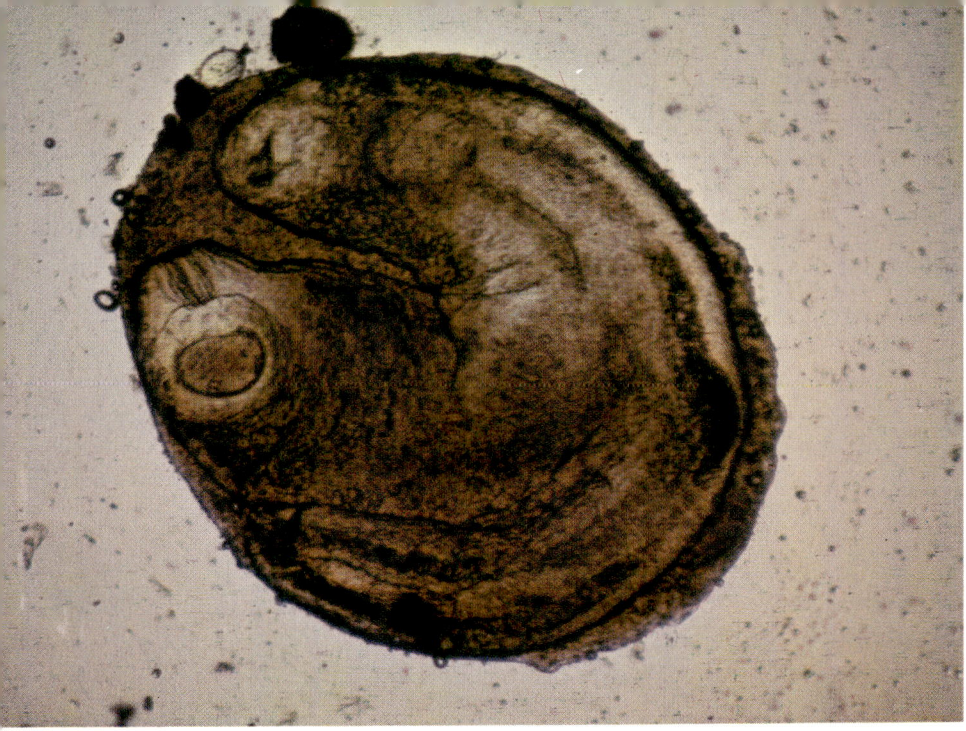

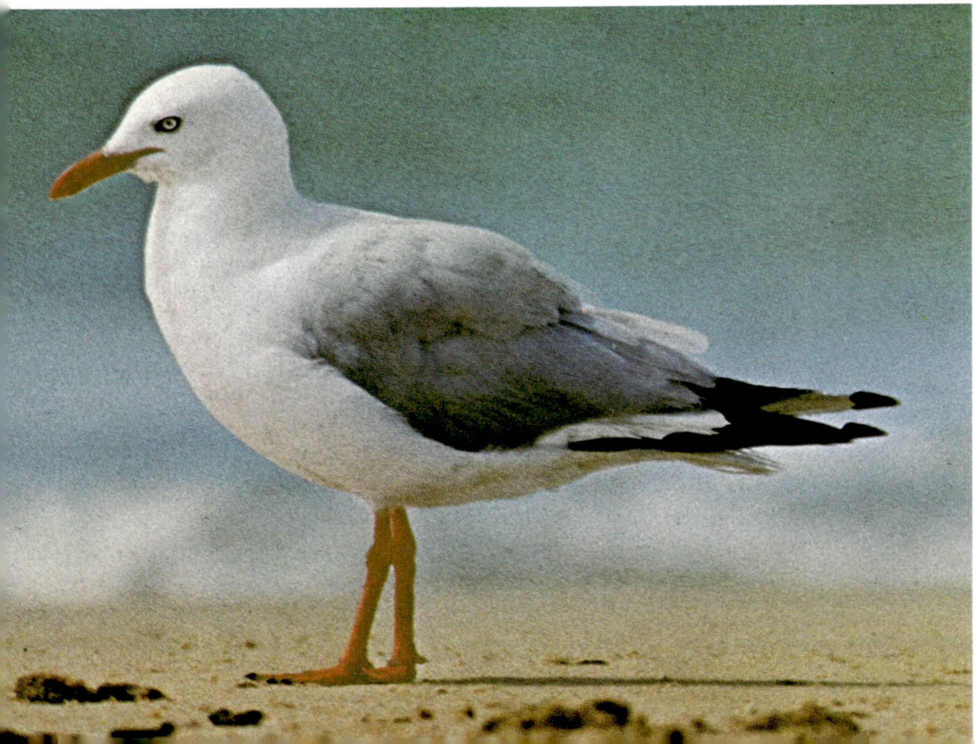

Many less common monogeneans have also been reported to infect marine fishes. Each species has the characteristic hooks, suckers and operculated filament-bearing eggs. For a more extensive description of the monogeneans affecting marine fishes, the specialized literature (64, 72) should be consulted.

Daitreosoma chaetodontis.
Left: adult worm.
Right: egg with filament.
After Reichenbach-Klinke.

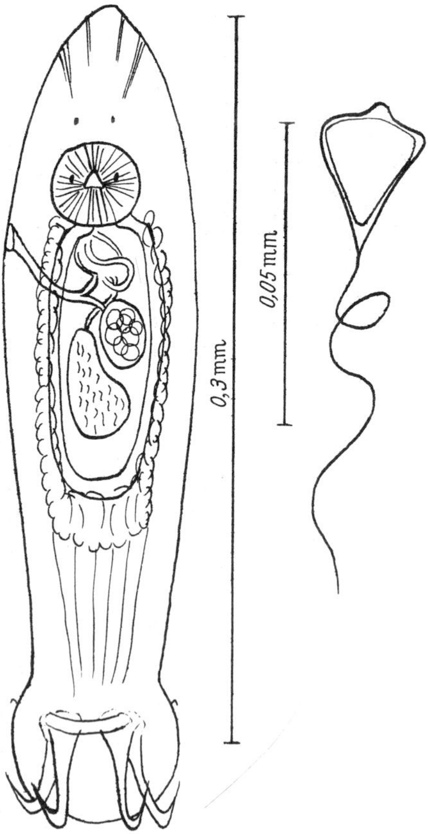

Diplectanum aculeatum.
After Sproston.

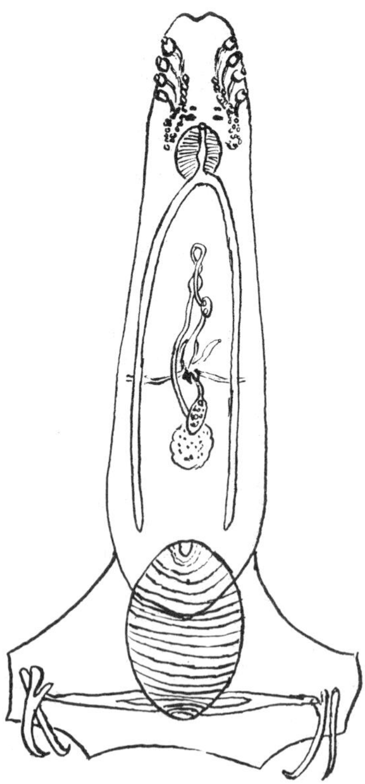

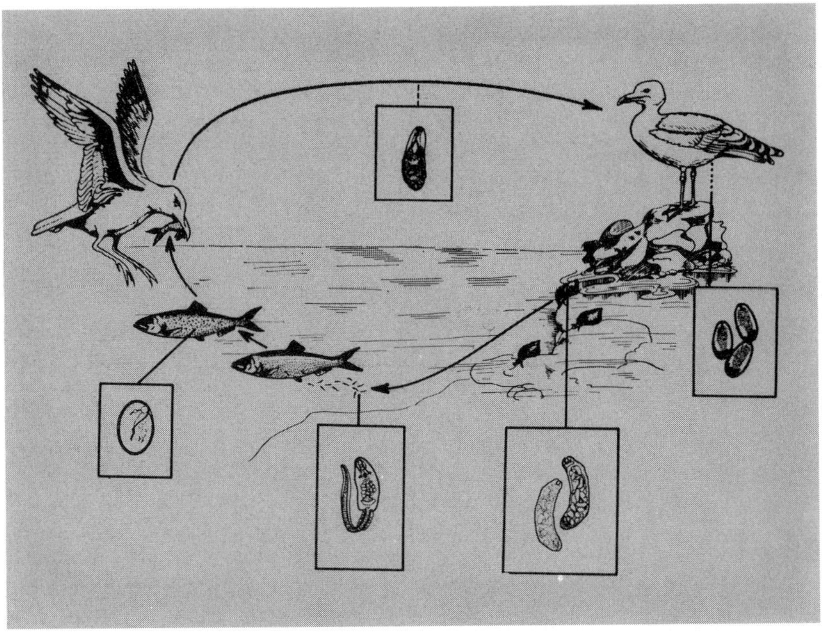

Life cycle of *Cryptocotyle lingua.* After Hoffman and Sindermann.

Digenetic Trematodes

Digenetic trematodes require an intermediate host, generally a snail. In some instances fishes are the final host for endoparasitic flukes, while at other times they serve as intermediate hosts, with the definitive stages occurring in fish-eating birds. Adult forms with two characteristic suckers may be found both in the intestine and circulatory system of fishes. Although intestinal flukes may shed eggs to further spread the parasite, they rarely cause mortalities by themselves. Among the blood-inhabiting species, egg masses have been associated with extensive damage to such vital organs as the kidney and heart.

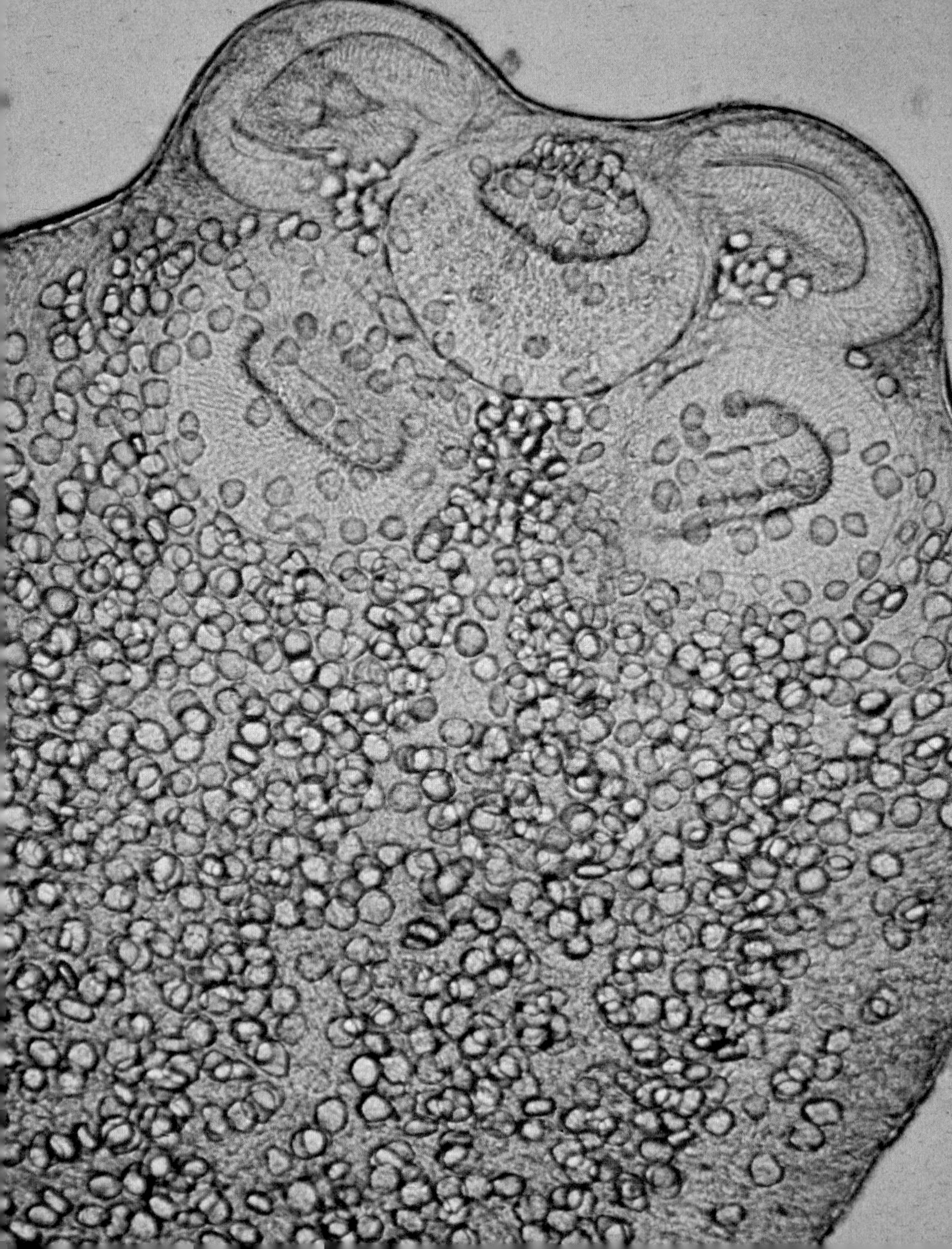

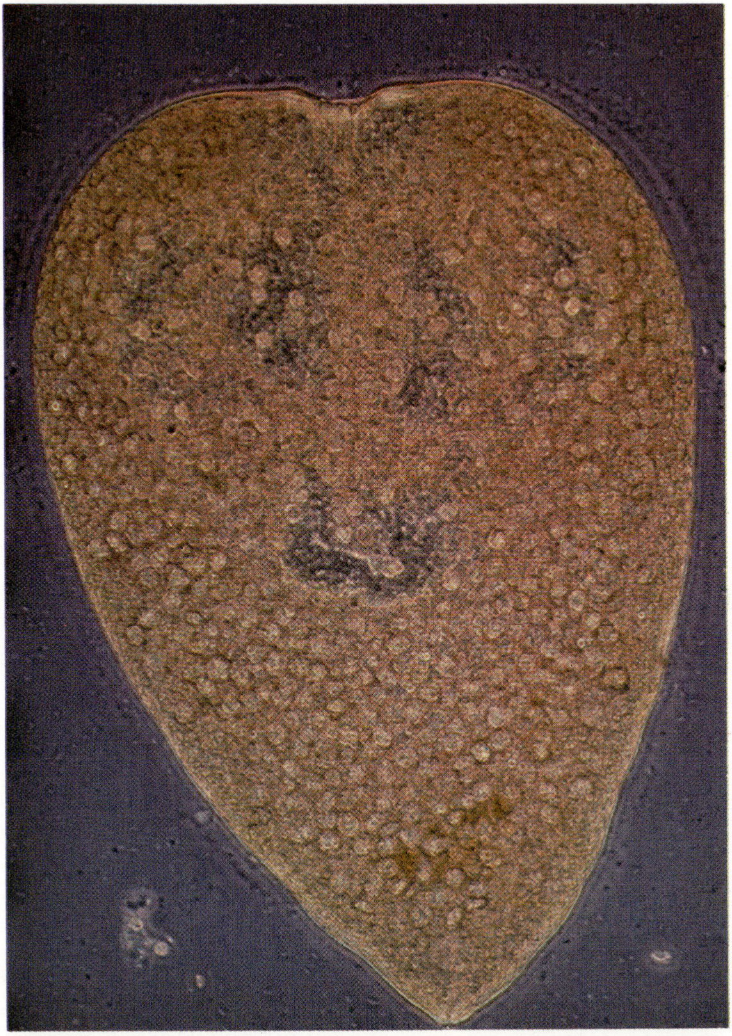

Above: This plerocercoid is from a tetraphyllidean tapeworm. Infected fishes can serve as a source of infection to predatory fishes, birds and mammals (including man). Photo by Frickhinger.

Opposite: The plerocercoid stage of tapeworm development has caused cystic lesions in a variety of tissues and organs. Most infected fishes have only one to four large-sized plerocercoids, but up to ten medium-sized larvae may sometimes be found. Photo by Frickhinger.

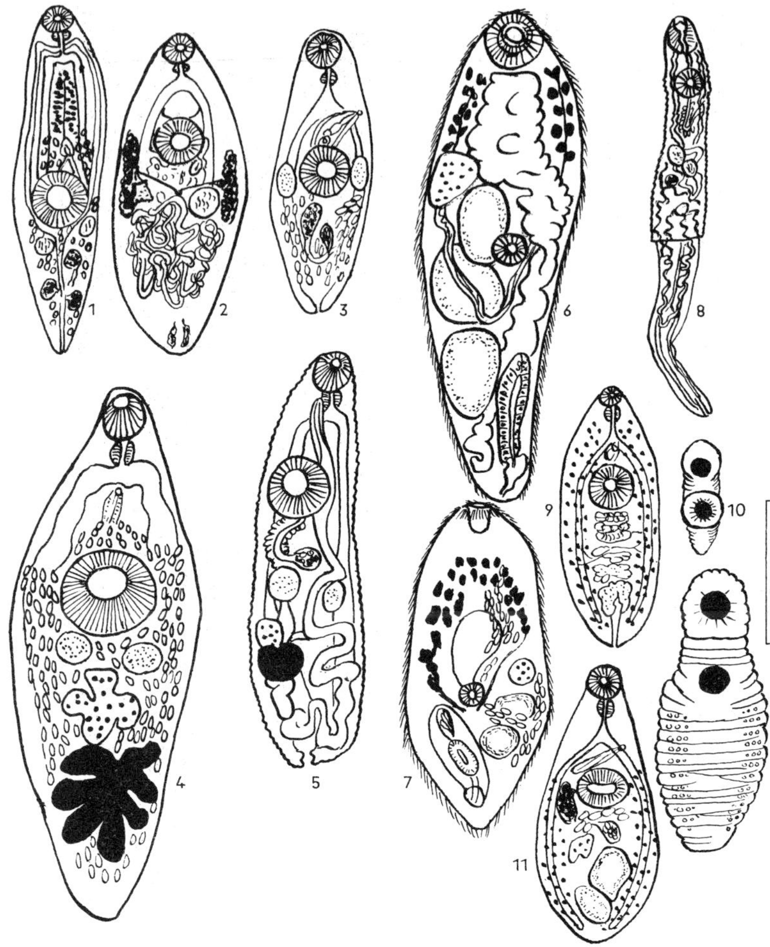

Digenetic trematodes from marine fishes. 1. *Derogenes varicus*, 2. *Steringaphorus furciger*, 3. *Zoogonoides viviparus*, 4. *Lecithaster gibbosus*, 5. *Aphanurus stossichi*, 6. *Bucephalopsis gracilescens*, 7. *Prosorhynchus crucibulum*, 8. *Lecithocladium excisium*, 9. *Helicometra fasciata*, 10. *Ptychogonimus megastomus* with juvenile specimen and 11. *Podocotyle atomon*. After Dawes.

Intermediate larval forms (metacercaria) have been found beneath the skin, within various internal organs or in the eye. When the eye is invaded, exophthalmia may occur. It is these larval forms which are associated with the most damage to host tissue. Metacercaria have caused occlusion of both hepatic and cardiac blood vessels. When these larval forms occur under the skin they are sometimes referred to as yellow grubs. These metacercaria are often surrounded by black pigment (black spot disease) and may bear spines. The extent of damage caused by digenetic trematode larvae depends upon the particular tissues being invaded.

CESTODES (TAPEWORMS)

Adult cestodes, or parasitic tapeworms, occur in the intestines of marine fishes, while intermediate stages occur in the flesh or liver. Fishes can become infected by eating small crustaceans (copepods) or tubificid worms that harbor infective stages. Infected fishes can serve as a source of infection to predatory fishes, birds or mammals (including man).

Trypanorhynchid tapeworms. 1. *Grillotia* sp., 2. *Lacistorhynchus tenuis*, 3. *Sphyriocephalus tergestinus*, 4. *Hepatoxylon trichiuri*, 5. *Nybelinia guenteri* and 6. larval *Tentacularia*. After Wardle-McLeod.

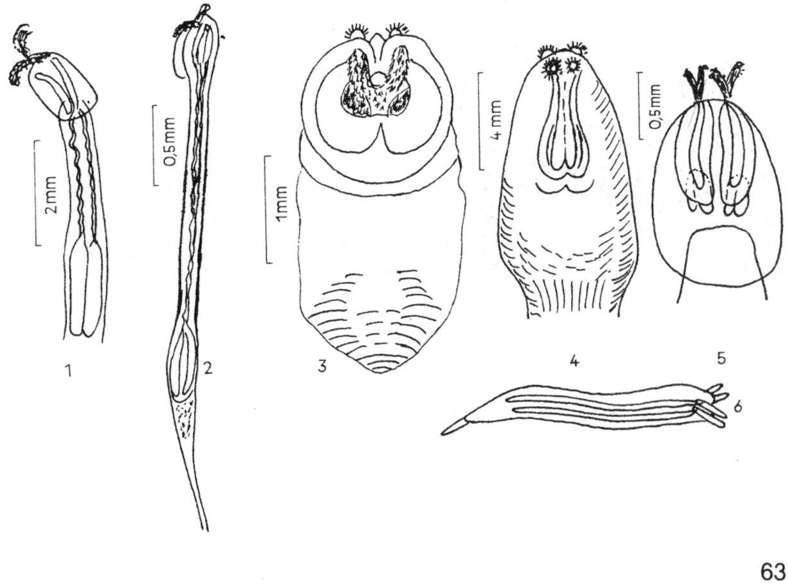

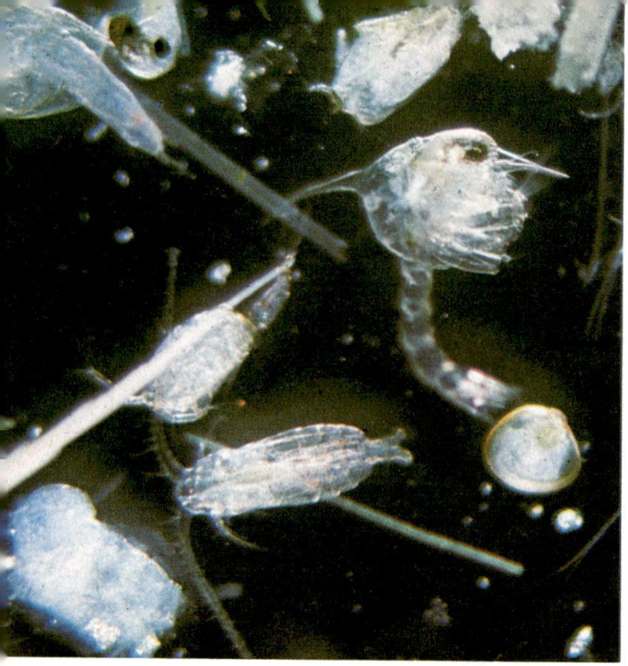

Marine zooplankton such as those shown at left are often consumed by marine fishes and may contain infective stages of cestodes. The cyclophyllidean tapeworm (*Amabilla* sp.) shown below is transmitted to fishes by copepods which act as intermediate hosts. Photo left by K. Gillett; photo below by Frickhinger.

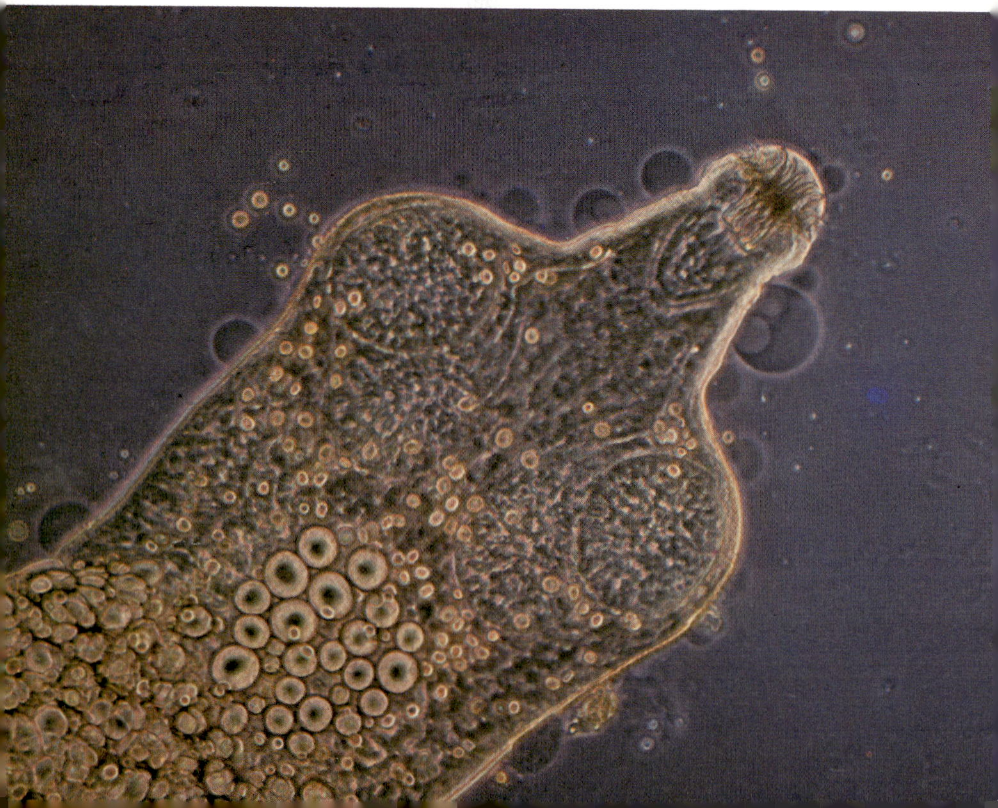

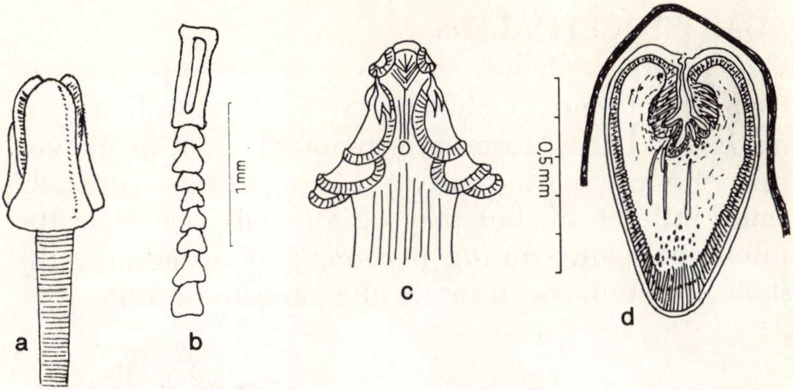

Tapeworms: a. *Ptychobothrium belones,* b. *Bothriocephalus scorpii* (after Wardle-McLeod), c. scolex of adult *Acanthobothrium coronatum* and d. larval form "Scolex pleuronectis" (after Reichenbach-Klinke).

Adult tapeworms are identified primarily on the basis of morphological characteristics of the scolex, which bears the attachment organs. The scolex may have acetabula (suckers), bothria (long, narrow sucking grooves), or bothridia (broad, leaf-like structures with thin, flexible margins). In addition to one or more of the above organs of attachment, cestodes parasitizing fishes usually also have anterior hooks and a body divided into numerous segments or proglottids. Many genera, including *Bothriocephalus*, *Agamonema*, *Eubothrium* and *Proteocephalus*, have been reported in *Fundulus* found in brackish waters.

As was the case with endoparasitic flukes, damage associated with tapeworm parasitism depends upon the extent of involvement in a particular tissue. The adult forms parasitizing the intestinal tract may debilitate the host or completely occlude the intestinal lumen. Typically, larval forms are much more damaging; they can infiltrate the liver, causing hepatic degeneration. Adult tapeworms can be effectively removed with small doses of Yomesan®

ACANTHOCEPHALIDS

Acanthocephalids, or thorny-headed worms, are frequently found attached to the intestinal wall of marine fishes. Larval forms are commonly seen in the viscera of many marine species. These parasites generally cause little harm, but they occasionally penetrate the intestinal wall, causing peritonitis. Crustaceans, the intermediate hosts, transmit the parasite to fishes.

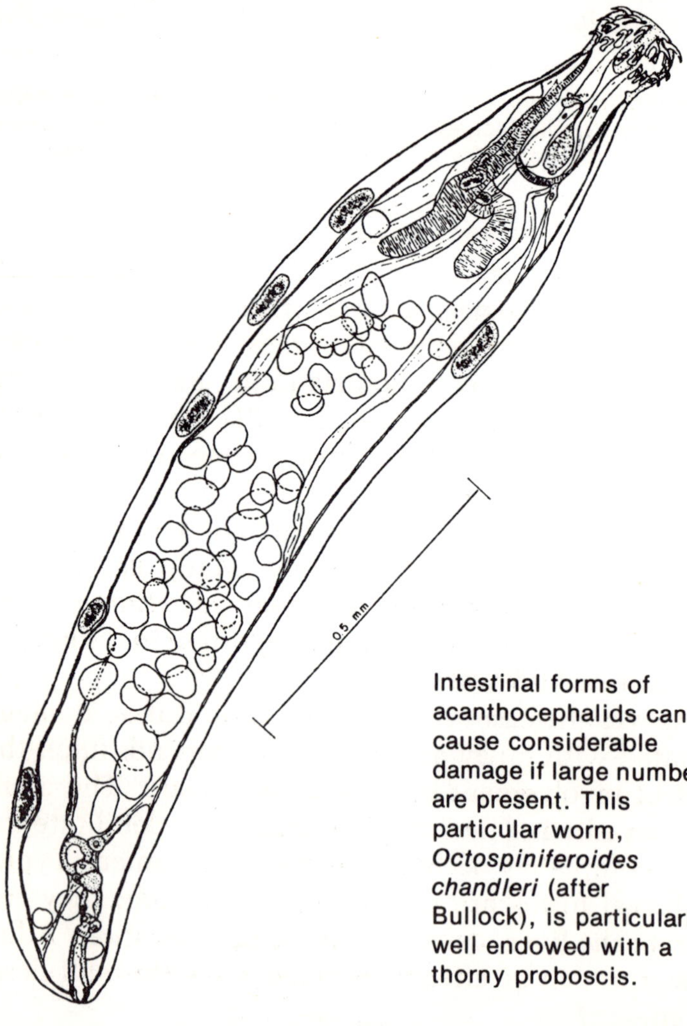

Intestinal forms of acanthocephalids can cause considerable damage if large numbers are present. This particular worm, *Octospiniferoides chandleri* (after Bullock), is particularly well endowed with a thorny proboscis.

NEMATODES (ROUNDWORMS)

The adult forms of parasitic nematodes are frequently found invading the intestinal lining or lying free in the abdominal cavity. Encysted larval stages have been observed in various body organs and body musculature. The final hosts of larval fish nematodes are piscivorous fishes, birds and mammals. These parasites can block the bile duct, damage the intestinal lining and otherwise cause harm to the host. Species which live within the circulatory system are transmitted by intermediate hosts such as copepods or free-living worms. Some of the more common genera of parasitic nematodes are *Contracaecum*, *Anisakis* and *Cucullanus*. Various anthelmintics have been successfully used for removing intestinal nematodes.

Life cycle of *Contracaecum aduncum*. 1. Sexually mature worm, 2. egg with embryo, 3. juvenile larva, 4. older larva. After Reichenbach-Klinke.

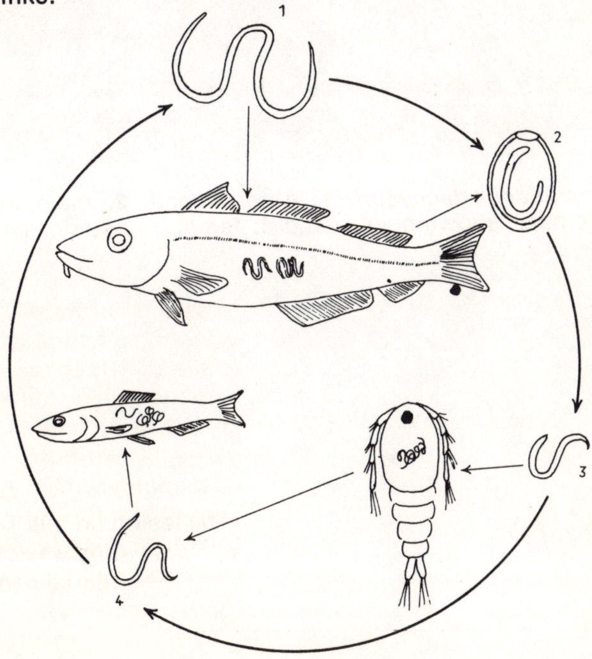

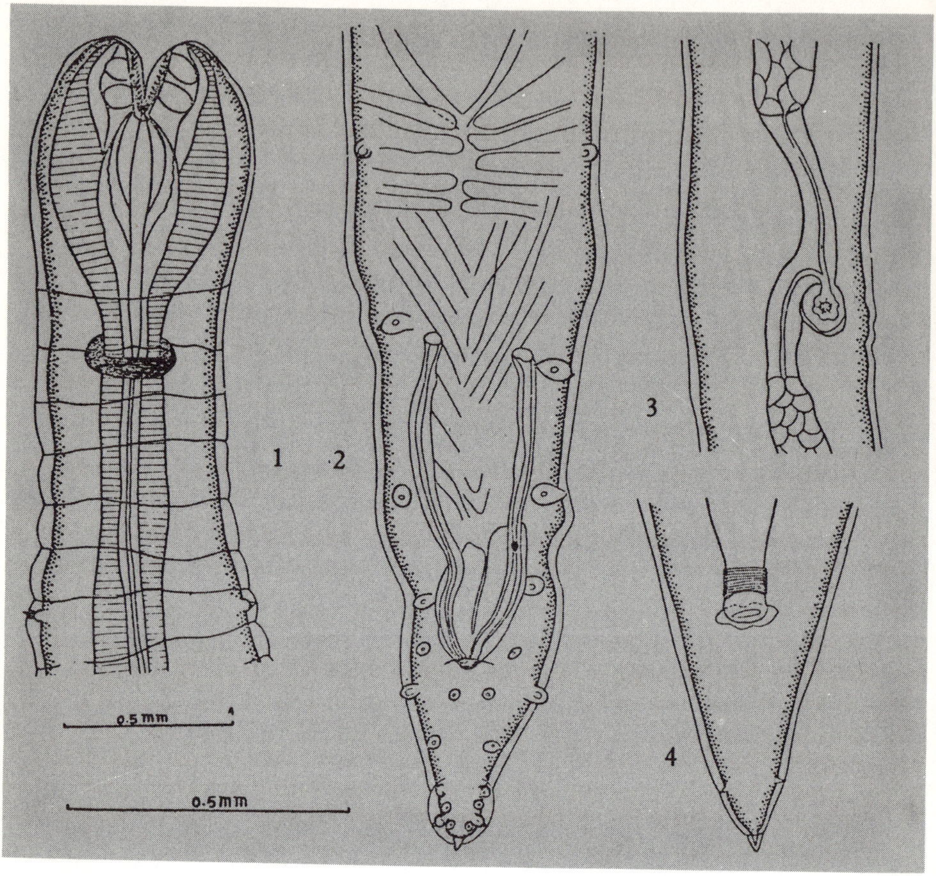

Pseudocucullanus tachysuri. 1. Anterior end, 2. male, posterior end, 3. female, showing vulva and 4. female, posterior end. After Margolis.

Opposite:
The lesion on this *Tetraodon fluviatilis* was caused by filarial nematodes.

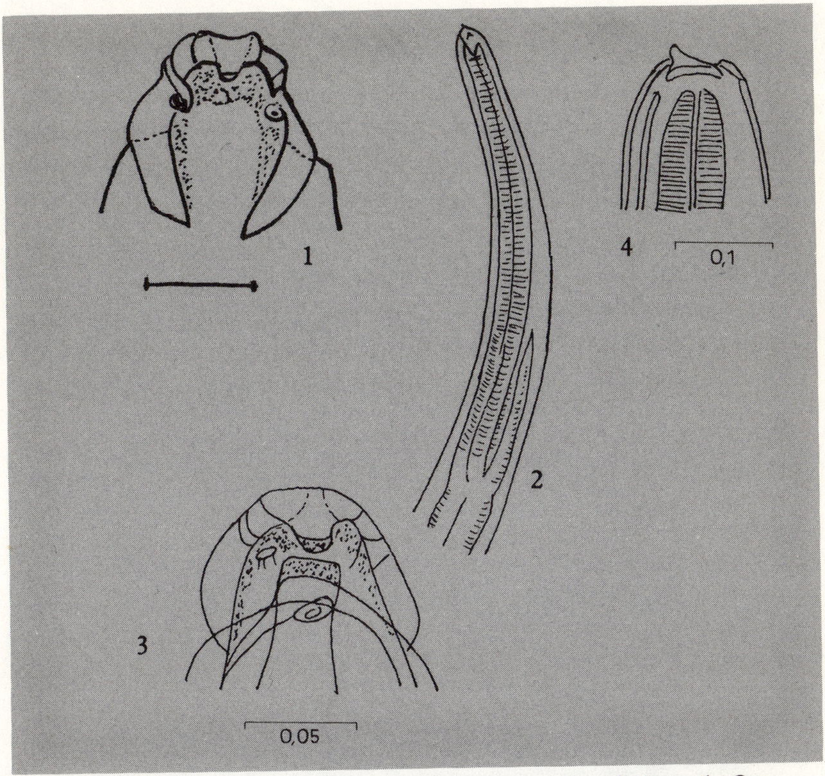

Anterior end of some nematodes parasitic to marine fishes. 1. *Contracaecum aduncum*, 2. *Porrocaecum reticulatum*, 3. *Rhaphidascaris acus* and 4. *Anisakis marina.* After Reichenbach-Klinke.

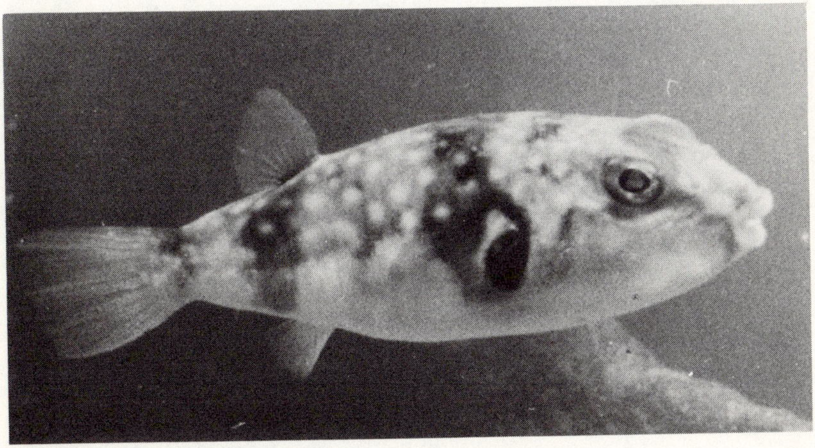

LEECHES

Leeches can cause harm to marine fishes not only by sucking blood from the host but also by acting in the transmission of *Cryptobia*, a flagellated blood parasite. The wounds left by various leeches often become the site of secondary bacterial infections. Leeches are not considered to be a problem in the marine aquarium, but they may be encountered in the collection of marine fishes from their native habitat. They can be effectively removed with a 5-second dip in lime solution (2 g lime/liter).

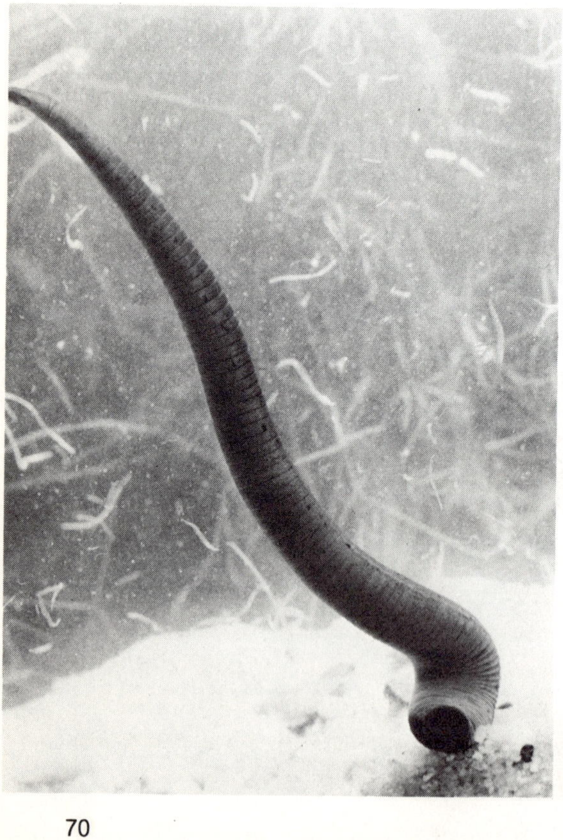

Leeches are occasionally encountered while collecting marine fishes. They can cause anemia, transmit disease and leave wounds which permit secondary bacterial invasion. Photo by Marcuse.

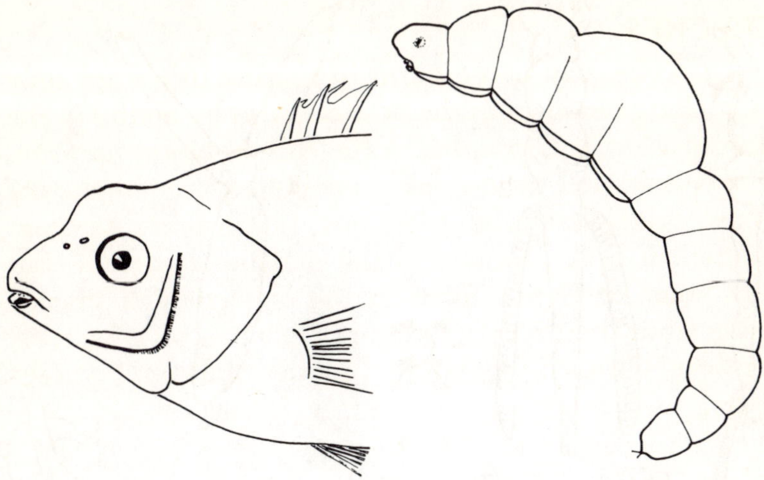

Head nodule (gibbosity) of *Centrolabrus exoletus* (left) found harboring the copepod *Leposphilus labrei* (right). After Quignard.

DISEASES CAUSED BY CRUSTACEANS

COPEPODS

Free-living copepods make up a significant portion of the marine zooplankton. Some of these marine copepods have lost their segmentation and extremities to become specialized external parasites of marine fishes. These parasites attach to the gills and body surfaces by means of claws at their anterior extremity or by special chitinous structures. Mouth parts (stylets) have become adapted to sucking nourishment from the host. Invasive species can cause severe dermal ulcerations, and the larger females can deplete the host of nourishment. *Caligus pageti* was reported to cause extensive losses among juvenile gray mullet, *Mugil capito* (56). The so-called "gibbosity" of some wrasses is due to a copepod living in the head of these fishes (43).

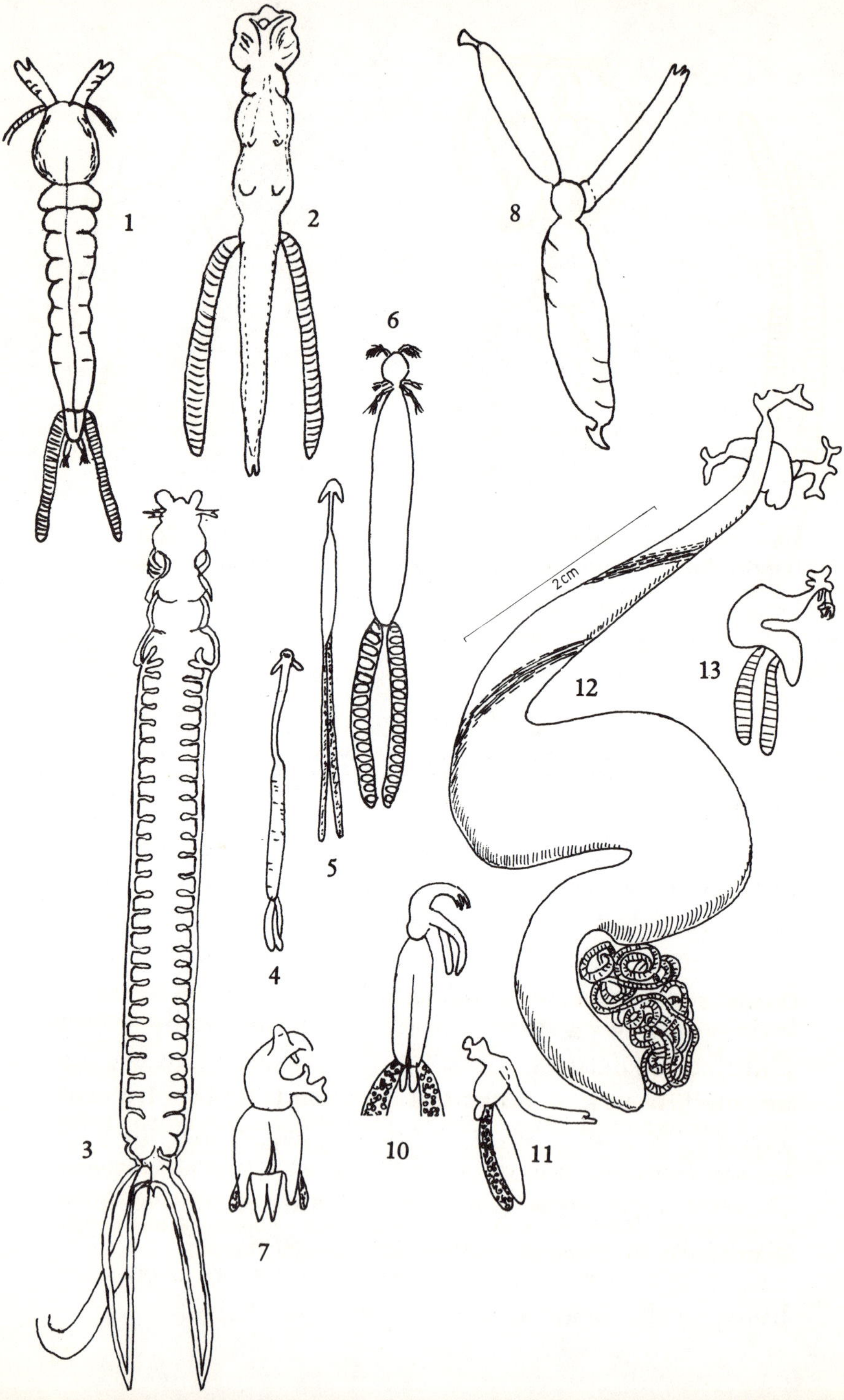
1
2
8
6
2cm
5
4
13
12
3
7
10
11

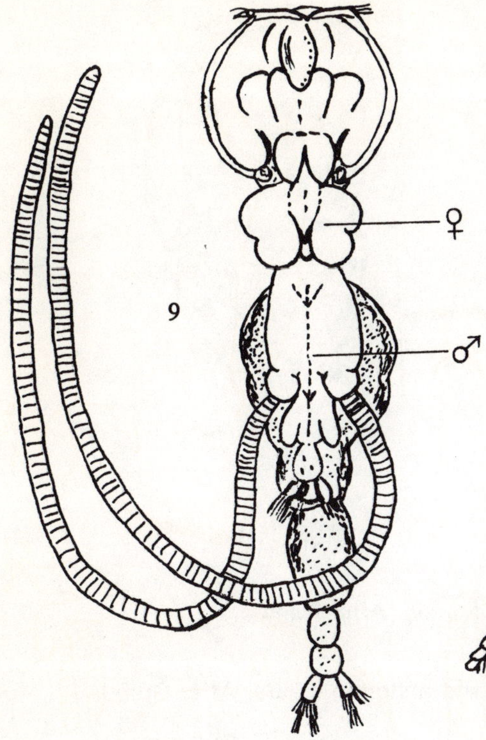

9

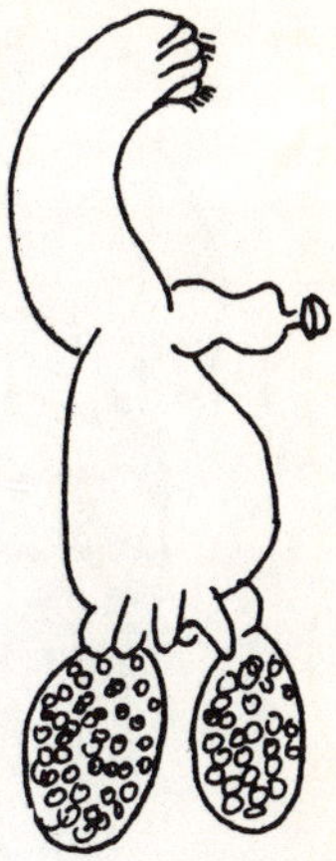

14

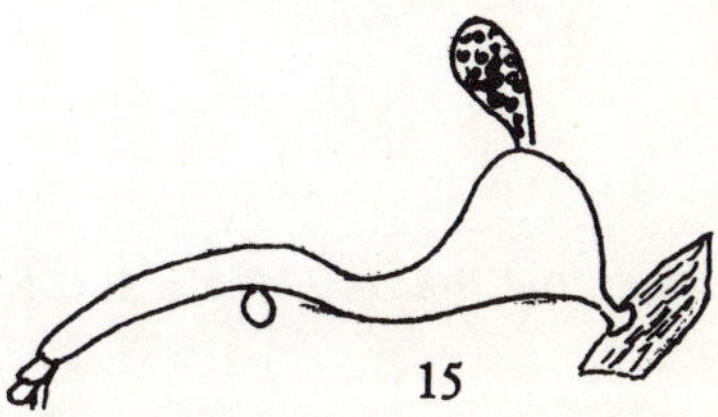

15

Opposite and above: Parasitic copepods from marine fishes. 1. *Dichelestium oblongum* (after Scott), 2. *Lamproglena pucchella* (after Markewitsch), 3. *Pseudocycnus thynnus* (after Brandes), 4. *Penella orthagorisci* (after Leigh-Sharpe), 5. *Lernaeenicus sprattae* (after Edwards), 6. *Hatschekia cornigera* (after Scott), 7. *Epibrachiella impudica* (after Scott), 8. *Tracheliastes polycolpus* (after v. Nordmann), 9. *Elythrophora brachyphora* (after Luling), 10. *Parabrachiella rostrata* (after Scott), 11. *Clavella scombri* (after Scott), 12. *Lernaeocera branchialis* (after Capart), 13. *Haemobaphes cyclopterina* (after Wilson), 14. *Brachiella obesa* (after Leigh-Sharpe) and 15. *Clavella sciatheri* (after Leigh-Sharpe).

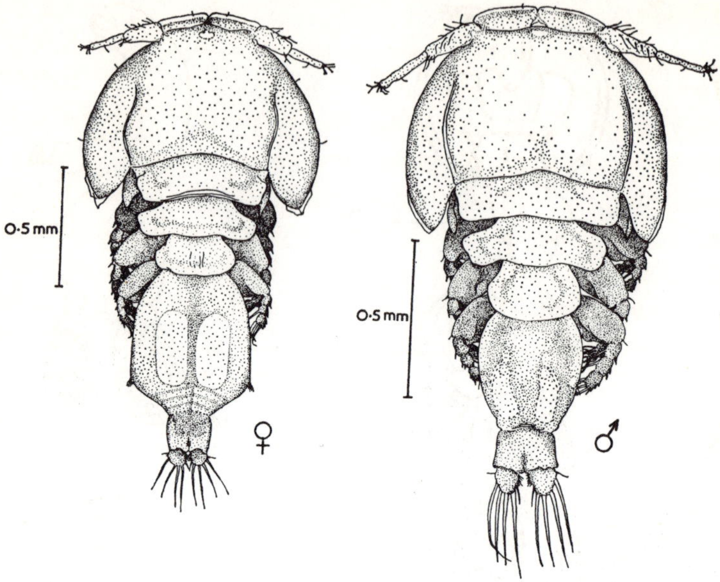

Dissonus manteri, male and female. After Kabata.

Cecrops latreilli from dorsal and abdominal side. After Grabda.

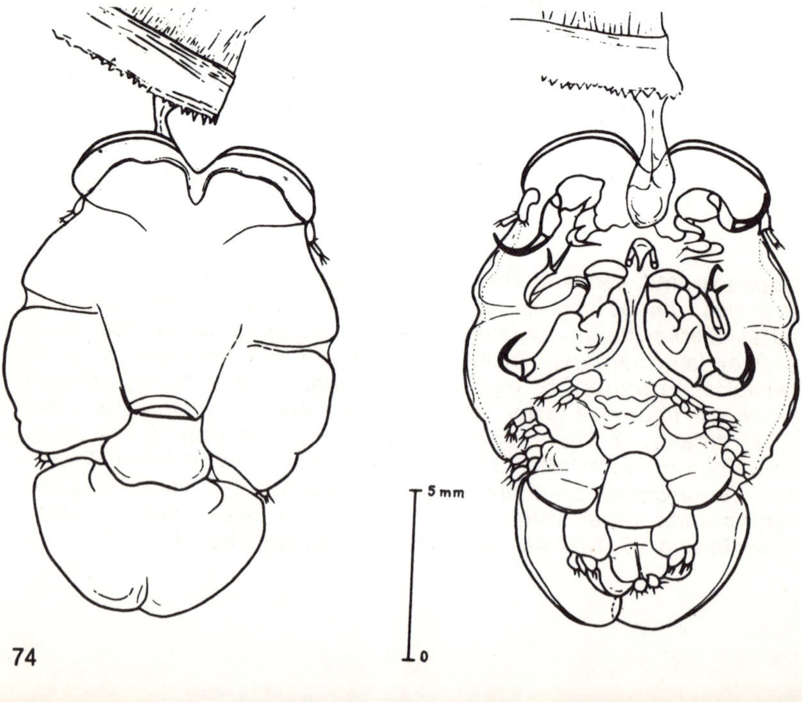

ISOPODS

Isopods are mostly free-living crustaceans, closely related to the decapods. Temporary parasitic forms attack marine fishes and whales. Frequently they attach to the base of fins with modified claw-like extremities. Nourishment is obtained by boring into the host's flesh. Parasitic isopods can debilitate a fish until its death. Because the parasites are so large, removing them by hand is preferred. In some cases it may be necessary to surgically remove the isopod; once the parasite has been removed, the wound should be disinfected.

Juvenile male of *Livoneca symmetrica.* After Reichenbach-Klinke.

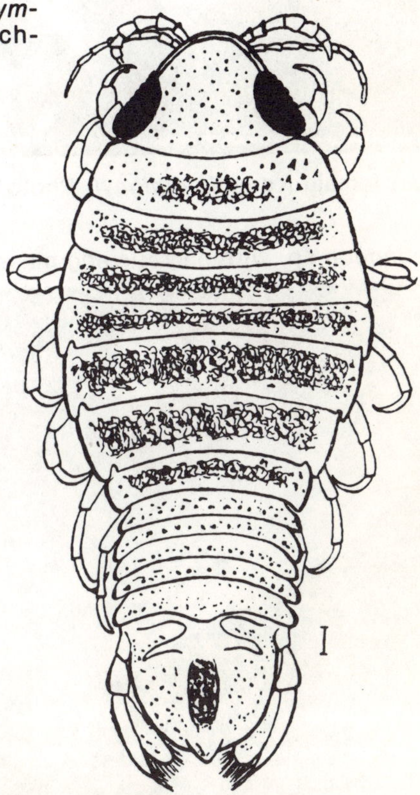

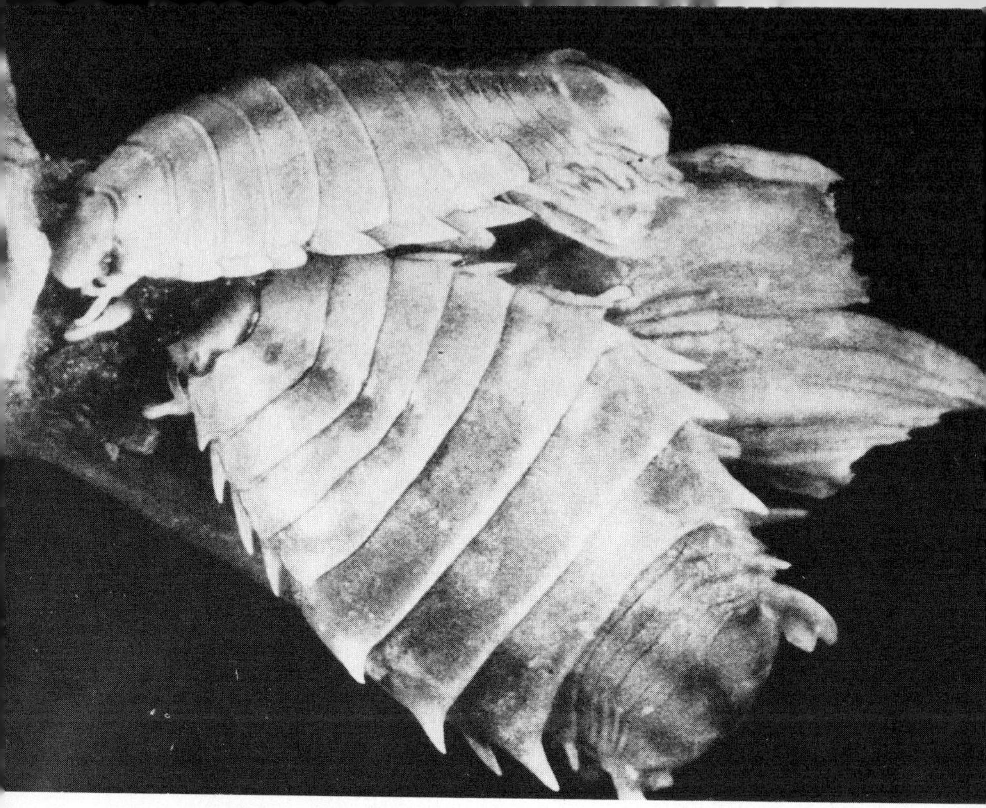

Two female *Nerocila orbignyi.* Photo by Wunder.

Tetraodon sp. with necrotic egg masses. Photo by Wossner.

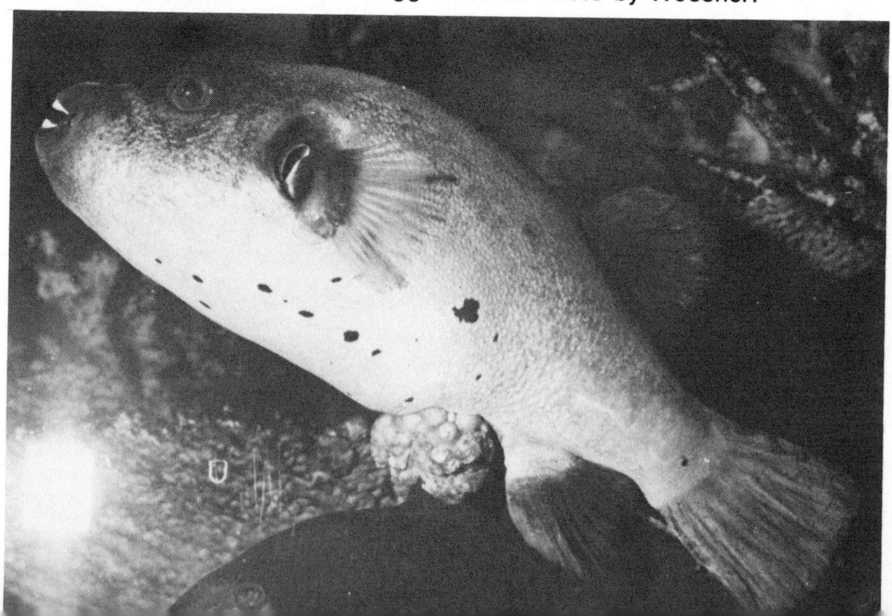

IV. Non-infectious Diseases

METABOLIC DISTURBANCES

Metabolic disturbances occur with much greater frequency in aquarium fishes than in wild fishes. By being deprived of their natural habitat, aquarium fishes often lack adequate swimming space and natural foods. The stress associated with captivity may result in a loss of appetite, emaciation and changes in the normal coloration of the fish. Many fishes maintained in marine aquariums are affected with various forms of liver damage including degeneration, lipoidosis, cirrhosis and finally necrosis. Twenty-one cases of liver degeneration caused largely by inadequate diet were reported in marine fishes kept in the New York Aquarium during a single year (35). When vitamin and mineral deficiencies are responsible for liver degeneration, feeding live foods can often reverse this condition. Nutritional imbalances can also lead to pathological changes in the kidney, spleen and ovaries. Infertility and an increased embryonic mortality may also occur.

One public aquarium reported that non-infectious diseases outnumbered infectious diseases (35). Generally non-infectious diseases stemmed from improper water chemistries, malnutrition and nitrogen supersaturation that resulted in gas emboli formation and subsequent death of the affected fishes. Gas bubble disease can occur when the water temperature is rapidly increased over a short period of time.

Fishes which survive the initial insult of a metabolic disturbance are more susceptible to secondary pathogenic invasion than are non-stressed fishes. Therefore, weakened survivors of a metabolic insult should receive particular attention with respect to nutrition, habitat and avoidance of further stress.

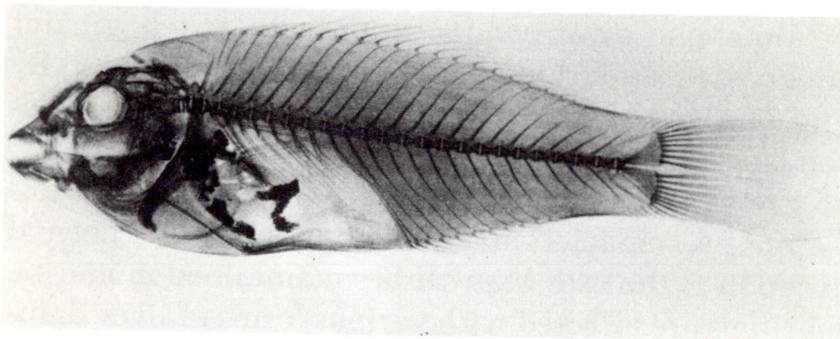

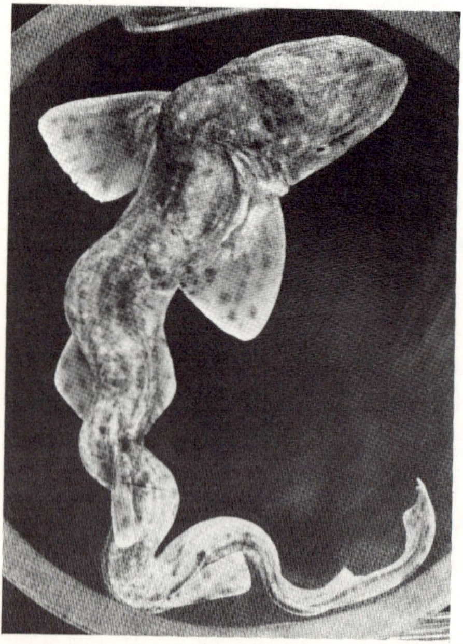

Above: Diagnostic radiography is occasionally used to detect pathological changes in fishes. This radiograph demonstrates normal skeletal development. Courtesy of Schindler. **Left:** This young dogfish shark, *Scylliorhinus canicula*, is affected with severe curvature of the spine. A variety of infectious and noninfectious diseases have been incriminated in causing skeletal deformations.

TUMORS, PSEUDOTUMORS AND SIMILAR HYPERTROPHIES

A variety of tumor-like lesions occur on marine fishes. Many of these are not tumors at all but parasitic cysts. Pseudotumors are swellings produced by a variety of parasites including myxosporidia, microsporidia and helminths. Rarely copepods can cause these tumor-like lesions. Multiple granulomas have been found in various body organs of marine fishes. Mycotic granulomas have been reported in the fishes' flesh (17). Fluid-filled cysts have been noted in the gall bladder, kidney and ovary; the exact cause was unknown.

Actual tumors of marine fishes have been reported in all body organs and tissues (17, 31, 57). Most of the

This white croaker, *Genyonemus lineatus*, is afflicted with an oral papilloma. Extensive growths such as this can severely impair normal feeding behavior. After Mawdesley-Thomas.

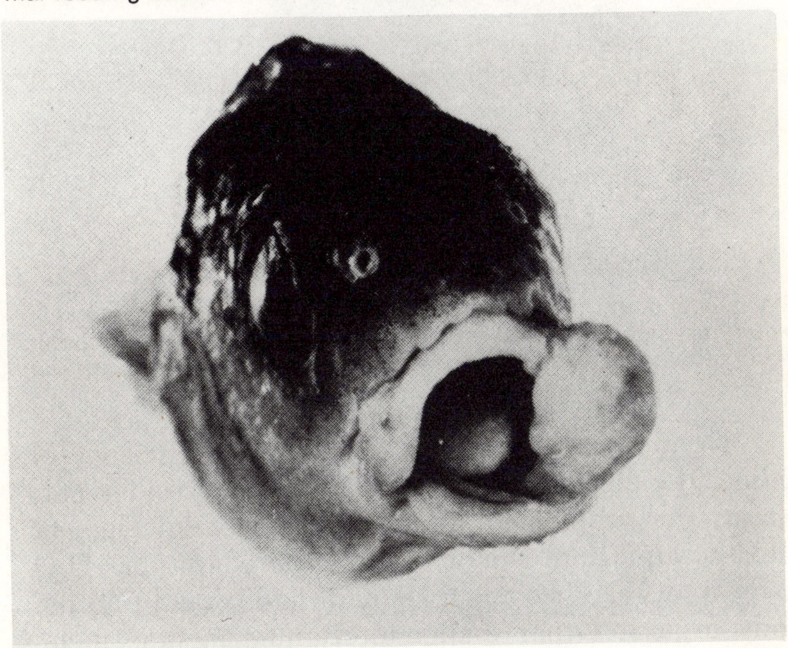

tumors affecting a fish's skin are either epitheliomas or papillomas (17). Tumors involving the blood system (hematomas and hemangiomas) are less common. Odontomas and ameloblastic fibro-odontomas have also been reported (17). Lipomas, which have frequently been reported in freshwater fishes, also occur in marine fishes. Fibromas also appear to be rather common (57), as are osteomas. Tumors of the nervous system (neuroblastomas and neurofibromas) are rare.

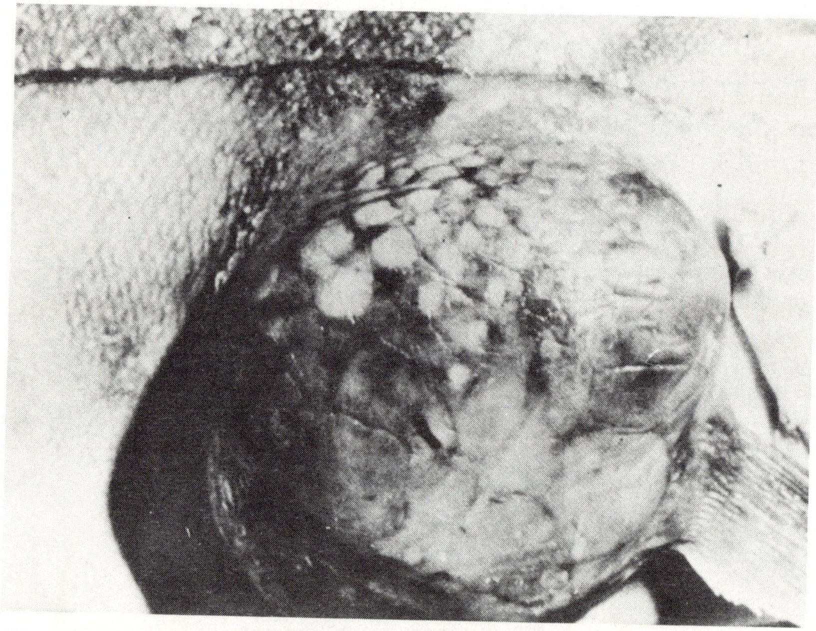

The lateral body musculature of this haddock, *Melanogrammus aeglefinus*, has developed an extensive yet well defined fibroma. Histopathological examination revealed the tumor to be composed of whorls of fibroblasts. After Mawdesley-Thomas.

Thyroid tumors can be caused by a deficiency of iodine. If iodine deficiency is the cause of thyroid hyperplasia, the supplementation of this essential element into the aquarium should reverse the condition. Thyroid tumors can become malignant and spread to other body organs. Other malignant tumors include melanomas of the skin and—less commonly—guanophoromas, lymphomas and neurofibrosarcomas.

The specific cause of tumors is generally not known. Papillomas are suspected of having a viral etiology, while other tumors may be hereditary or environmentally induced.

DEVELOPMENTAL ABNORMALITIES

Many different developmental abnormalities have been reported in marine fishes, although the reports are much less numerous than those given for freshwater fishes. These anomalies include skeletal deformities, fin malformations and abnormal sexual development. Although sex changes (protandric development) and hermaphroditism are normal in many marine species, these conditions have also been reported in species in which they are considered to be departures from the normal.

This skeletal drawing of a marine fish demonstrates several osteomas. After Bell, from Mawdesley-Thomas.

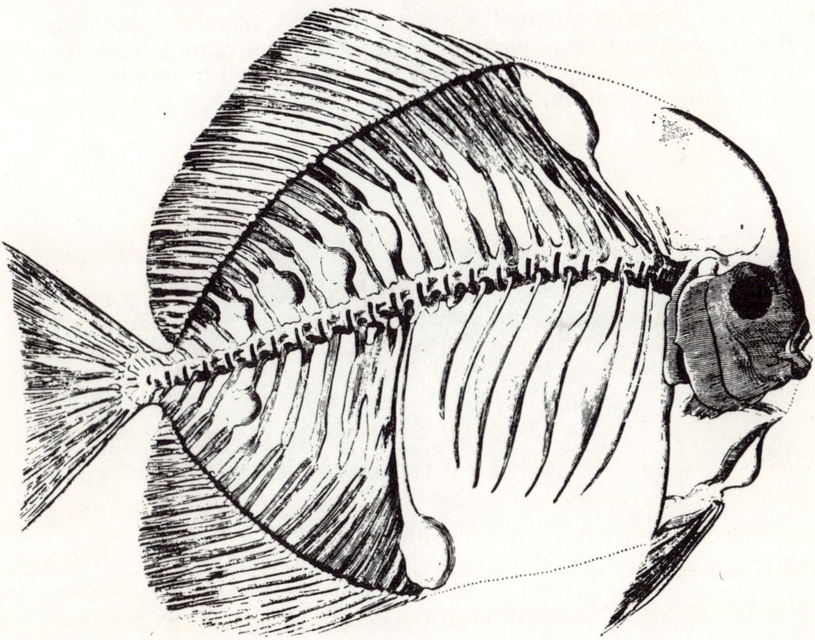

DAMAGES DUE TO ENVIRONMENTAL FACTORS

Abnormal environmental conditions such as lack of oxygen, adverse water temperature, nitrogen supersaturation, heavy metal poisoning and excessive buildup of metabolic waste products have been responsible for numerous mortalities among marine fishes. Direct poisoning can be caused either by the ingestion of toxic foods or by secretions from poisonous fishes and algae.

Environmental stress has been shown to increase a fish's susceptibility to disease, so stress-related factors such as keeping incompatible species together in the same tank should be avoided. Conscientious daily observation of the fishes' behavior, coupled with monitoring the water quality, will greatly help the aquarist in the early detection of disease. Once diagnosed, mortalities can generally be avoided by prompt corrective measures or specific therapy.

Should an aquarist suspect a disorder of the skeletal system, a radiograph should be requested. Most veterinary clinics have the capability to radiograph fishes. The skeletal system of this marine fish is normal. Courtesy of Schindler.

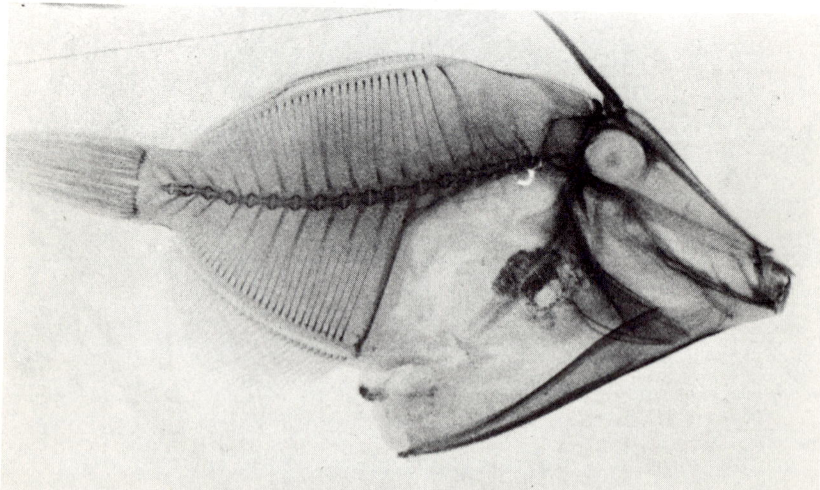

V. Treatment of Diseases

The first step an aquarist should take after recognizing an abnormality in fish behavior should be to check out the various aquarium equipment. Malfunctions in heating, lighting, filtration, and aeration equipment can lead to adverse environmental conditions. The water quality parameters such as dissolved oxygen, pH, salinity, ammonia nitrogen levels and general cleanliness of the tank should also be investigated. If environmental conditions appear optimal the fish should then be closely observed for the presence of skin parasites or wounds. If mortalities occur, the gills and internal organs should be examined for the presence of parasites and pathological changes. It may be necessary to send diseased fishes to a special institution for diagnosis. This must be done immediately; only fresh specimens show the clinical signs necessary for an accurate diagnosis.

Strengthening the fishes' normal resistance by feeding natural foods or supplemental vitamins may be sufficient to alleviate the disease; fishes are capable of developing a natural immunity to a variety of infectious diseases.

Therapeutic agents are necessary to bring about a full recovery in the case of some infectious diseases. The appropriate therapeutic can be selected only after a definitive diagnosis has been made. A wide variety of antibiotics and sulfonamids have been successfully used to treat bacterial diseases of marine fishes.

Fungal infections can be treated with griseofulvin or malachite green. Ectoparasites have been treated successfully with copper sulfate, chloroquine, trichlorfon and formalin. *Hexamita* can be effectively destroyed with Flagyl®. Parasites of internal organs are difficult to treat. Sporozoans, myxosporidia and microsporidia, like internal fungi, cannot be reached by conventional methods. In these cases the diseased fishes should be eliminated. Piperazine can be used to control roundworm parasitism; Yomesan® (niclosamide) works well for treating tapeworm parasitism.

Because of the tremendous diversity of marine fishes, specific dosages of medicaments can vary. When many fishes are diseased, it is advisable to test the therapeutic agent on a few isolated individuals before treating all fishes.

COMMONLY USED THERAPEUTICS FOR FISH DISEASES

As an aid to suppliers desiring to locate these therapeutics, the name and address of an American manufacturer has been listed for most products. In most cases, individuals cannot obtain drugs or chemicals directly from the manufacturer. Most of these therapeutic agents are not approved by the Food and Drug Administration for use in fishes. The manufacturers listed do not necessarily endorse the prescribed uses, procedures or dosages. Under no circumstances shall the manufacturer, author, or publisher be considered liable to any person for any damage resulting from reliance on the information contained herein.

Certain of the listed drugs are available through normal fish hobby supply channels (pet shops, tropical fish stores, etc.) because they have been incorporated into commercially formulated remedies intended to combat specific ailments. These medications are obtainable economically and without prescription and of course have the additional value of being formulated in strengths easily applicable to aquarium usage.

BACTERIAL DISEASES:

Aureomycin® (chlortetracycline): 1 to 2 g/kg in the food over a 10-day period. Aureomycin® is manufactured by American Cyanamid Co., Agricultural Division, P.O. Box 400, Princeton, NJ 08540.

Betadine® (iodophor): 25 ppm for up to 5 min bath. Betadine® is manufactured by the Perdue Frederick Co., Norwalk, CT 06856.

Chloromycetin® (chloramphenicol): 6 to 11 mg/liter tank water for 5 to 7 days. Chloromycetin® is manufactured by Parke, Davis and Co., P.O. Box 118, Detroit, MI 48232.

Furacin® (nitrofurazone): 0.01% in the food for 1-2 weeks. Furacin® preparations are manufactured by Norden Laboratories, Inc., Lincoln NB 68501.

Furanace® (nifurpirinol): 3.8 mg per 10 gal tank water. Furanace® is manufactured by the Veterinary Products Div., Abbott Laboratories, North Chicago, IL 60064. Furanace® is marketed for aquarium use and is available at most pet shops.

Furoxone® (furazolidone): 25 mg/kg body weight for 10 days. Furoxone® preparations are manufactured by Norden Laboratories, Inc., Lincoln, NB 68501.

Kantrim® (kanamycin sulfate): Intraperitoneal injection 0.02 mg/g of fish against myxobacterial infections. Kantrim® is manufactured by the Veterinary Products Div., Bristol Laboratories, Syracuse, NY 13201.

Sulfa drugs: Various sulfonamides are used to treat fish diseases. Singly, or in combination with other sulfa drugs, the dosage is 16-20 g of sulfa drug(s) per 100 kg of fish, in the food. Sulfa-24® (sulfamethazine, sulfathiazole, sulfapyridine) is manufactured by Bio-Ceutic Laboratories, P.O. Box 999, St. Joseph, MO 64502. Sulfaguanidine is manufactured by Med-Tech Inc., P.O. Box 338, Elwood, KS 66024. Bactrim® (sulfamethoxazole) and Gantrisin® (sulfisoxazole) are manufactured by Roche Chemical Div., 340 Kingsland Road, Nutley, NJ 07110. Sulfamerazine fish grade is manufactured by American Cyanamid Co., Agriculture Division, P.O. Box 400, Princeton, NJ 08540.

Terramycin® (oxytetracycline): 1.8 mg/g of food, or by injection, 3 mg/150-400 g fish. Terramycin® products are manufactured by Pfizer Inc., 235 42nd Street, New York, NY 10017.

ECTOPARASITES:

Ammonia: Use 1:1,000 to 1:2,000 of a 10% commercial solution for a 5 to 10 minute bath.

Aureomycin® (chlortetracycline): 0.5 to 0.6 mg/l against protozoans.

Chloroquine phosphate (Aralen® phosphate): Using a 1% stock solution, add 3 cc/liter of water. Aralen is manufactured by Winthrop Laboratories, 90 Park Avenue, New York, NY 10016.

Copper sulfate: 0.15 ppm for 14 days, used against *Oodinium.* Commercially prepared copper sulfate solutions are available at most pet shops.

Formalin: Using a 1% stock solution, add 2 cc/liter of water. Formalin can be purchased from scientific supply houses (Fisher Scientific Co., 203 Fisher Bldg., Pittsburg, PA 15219). Small quantities may be obtained from a local mortuary.

Methylene blue (methyl thionine chloride—not to be confused with methyl blue): Using a 1% stock solution (1 g/100 cc) add 3 to 6 drops /liter of water. Methblu® is manufactured by Haver-Lockhart Laboratories, P.O. Box 390, Shawnee Mission, KS 66201. Methylene blue solutions are also commercially available for aquarium use at most pet stores.

Salicylic acid: Using a 1% stock solution, add 10 cc/liter of water. Available from chemical supply houses.

Trichlorfon: 1 ppm added to the tank water, may be repeated once weekly for 3 treatments. As a bath use 25 ppm for 5 minutes. Trichlorfon is a contact insecticide, available at plant supply stores and livestock outlets under a variety of trade names such as Dipterex, Dylox, Dyrex, Chlorphos, Bot-X, Masoten, and Neguvon.

FUNGI:

Betadine® (iodophor): 25 ppm/5 min bath.

Griseofulvin (Fulvicin-U/F®): 10 mg/liter of water for treatment of internal fungi. Fulvicin-U/F® is manufactured by Schering Corporation, Galloping Hill Rd., Kenilworth, NJ 07033.

Malachite green: Using a 1% stock solution, add 10 cc/liter of tank water. Malachite green crystals are available from various chemical and biological supply houses. Commercially prepared solutions are available at pet stores.

Roccal® (benzalkonium chloride): 25 ppm for up to 5 min bath. Roccal® is manufactured by Winthrop Laboratories, 90 Park Ave., New York, NY 10016.

INTERNAL PARASITES:

Dibutyl tin oxide (biocidal rubber): 250 mg/kg of feed, fed over a 5 day period for removal of intestinal tapeworms, acanthocephalids.

Flagyl® (metronidazole): 1% medicated food over 5 to 7 days for *Hexamita* infections. Flagyl® is manufactured by Searle and Co., San Juan, Puerto Rico 00936.

Niclosamide (Yomesan®, Fenasal®, Mansonil®): 50 mg/10 g dried food for cestodes. Yomesan® is manufactured by Haver-Lockhart Laboratories, P.O. Box 390, Shawnee Mission, KS 66201.

VIRAL DISEASES:

There are no therapeutics proven to be effective against viral diseases of fishes. Various iodophors have been used although their effectiveness is questionable. The development of immunizing agents for both viral and bacterial pathogens is still in the experimental phase; however, the two-step infusion method shows much promise in this regard. The infusion method of immunizing fishes involves placing the fish in a hypertonic sodium chloride solution for 2 minutes, then transferring them into an antigen bath.

VI. Relationship of Fish Diseases to Human Diseases

Although marine aquarium fishes can harbor infectious agents which are pathogenic to man, the chances of an aquarist's becoming infected are remote. Fish cestodes and nematodes can be transmitted to man only when the fish is eaten raw, so an infection with tapeworms or roundworms poses no threat to an aquarist. There are no reports of fishes harboring viruses which are pathogenic to man. Shellfishes have been known to contain the virulent hepatitis virus, but this is not considered to be a problem in the marine aquarium.

There have been isolated reports of humans acquiring mycobacterially induced skin infections after handling fishes suffering from piscine tuberculosis. *Mycobacterium fortuitum* is a human pathogen, and *M. marinum* is suspect; both of these organisms are capable of growth at 37° C.

People who became infected with *M. fortuitum* had skin lesions at the time their hands were placed in the aquarium; apparently the bacteria are incapable of invading healthy skin. Aquarists with skin lesions should not place their hands in the aquarium; if it is necessary to handle fishes, protective gloves should be worn.

Fishes can also be asymptomatic carriers of the human pathogen *Escherichia coli* and various *Salmonella* and *Shigella;* however, there are no reports of persons having become infected with these organisms after handling aquarium fishes. Bacteria in the genus *Vibrio* are known to infect both marine fishes and man. Although it is unlikely that an aquarist would become infected with these potential human pathogens, caution should always be exercised when handling fishes. As a preventive measure, aquarists should always wash their hands and lower arms after exposing them to aquarium water.

Perhaps the greatest threat to the uninformed aquarist relates to the handling of venomous fishes such as *Pterois.* The venom apparatus of scorpionfishes and other venomous species is contained within various spines, particularly those in the dorsal fin. Over 200 species of marine fishes have been reported to be venomous; some of these are commonly kept by marine aquarists. Venomous fishes should be handled only when necessary and then with due caution. A physician should be consulted should the aquarist unwittingly become stung by a venomous marine fish.

Although striking in appearance, this lionfish, *Pterois* sp., can inflict a painful sting to the uninformed aquarist who might unwittingly handle it. Photo by Marcuse.

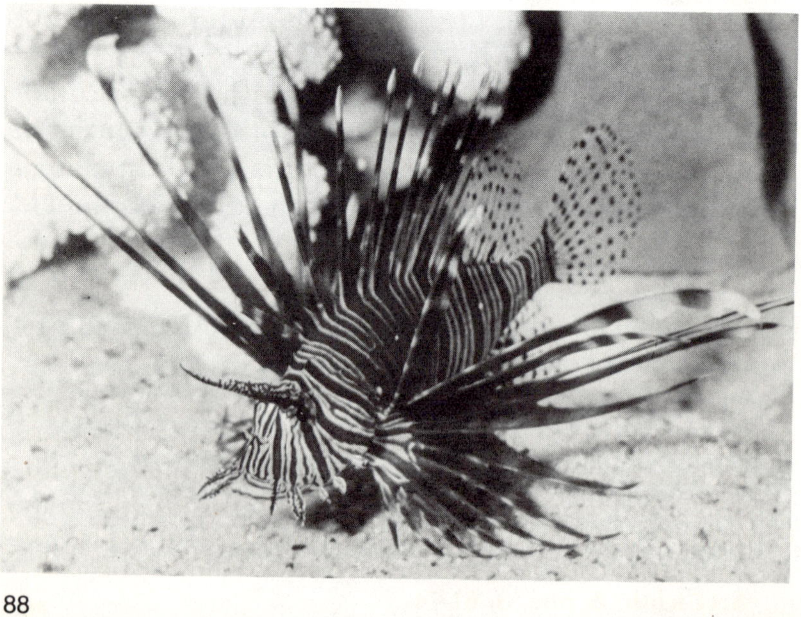

References

1. Aleem, A.A., M. Ruivo and J. Theodorides. 1953. Un cas de maladie a Saprolegniale chez une Atherina des environs de Salses. Vie et milieu 3: 44-51.
2. Alexandrowicz, J.S. 1952. Lymphocystis tumors in the red mullet (*Mullus surmuletus*). J. Mar. Biol. Ass. UK 30: 315-332.
3. Aronson, J.D. 1926. Spontaneous tuberculosis in saltwater fish. J. Infect. Dis. 39: 315-320.
4. Brown, E.M. 1934. On *Oodinium ocellatum*, a parasitic dinoflagellata causing epidemic disease in marine fish. Proc. Zool. Soc. London. 583-607.
5. Brown, E.M. 1951. *Cryptocaryon irritans* gen. et sp. n. Proc. Zool. Soc. London 120. Agenda and Abstracts, Scient. Meet. 11: 1-2.
6. Brown, E.M. and R. Hovasse. 1946. *Amyloodinium ocellatum*, a peridinean parasite on marine fishes. A complementary study. Proc. Zool. Soc. London. 116: 33-46.
7. Bullock, W.L. 1957. *Octospiniferoides chandleri* n. gen., n. sp., Neoechinorhynchid Acanthocephalan from *Fundulus grandis* Baird and Girard on the Texas coast. J. Paras. 43: 97-100.
8. Bullock, G.L., D.A. Conroy and S.F. Snieszko. 1971. Bacterial Diseases of Fishes, Vol. 2 A. T.F.H. Publications, Neptune City, N.J.
9. Clem, L.W., M. Sigel and R. Friis. 1965. An orphan virus isolated in marine fish cell tissue culture. Ann. N.Y. Acad. Sci. 126: 343-361.
10. Conroy, D.A. 1963. Un caso de putrefaccion de la aleta caudal observado en la corvina. Inst. Biol. mar. cienc. Inves. 19: 333.
11. Conroy, D.A. 1963. Studies on the application of Kanamycin to the control and treatment of some bacterial fish diseases. J. Appl. Bact. 26: 82-192.
12. Dillon, W.A. 1966. Provisional list of parasites occurring on *Fundulus* spp. Virginia J. 17: 21-31.
13. Duijn, C. van. 1973. Diseases of Fishes. 3 edit. Iliffe, London.
14. Ferguson, H.W. and R.J. Roberts. 1975. Myeloid leucosis associated with sporozoan infection in cultured Turbot (*Scophthalmus maximus*). J. Comp. Path. 85: 317-326.
15. Grabda, J. 1973. Contribution to knowledge of biology of *Cecrops latreillii*, the parasite of the ocean sunfish *Mola mola*. Acta ichth. & pisc. 3: 61-74.

16. Guiart, J. 1938. Etude parasitologique et epidemiologique de quelques poissons de mer. Bull. Inst. Oceanogr. Monaco. 775: 1-15.
17. Harshbarger, J.C. 1975. Registry of Tumors in lower animals. Activities Report, Mus. Nat. Hist., Smithsonian Inst. Washington, D.C.
18. Henley, M.W. and D.H. Lewis. 1976. Anaerobic Bacteria Associated with Epizootics in Grey Mullet (*Mugil cephalus*) and Redfish (*Sciaenops ocellata*) along the Texas Gulf Coast. J. Wildlife Dis. 12: 448-453.
19. Kabata, Z. 1966. Copepoda parasitic on Australian Fishes. V. Genus *Dissonus* (Dissonidae). Ann. Mag. Nat. Hist., ser. 13, 9: 211-266.
20. Kalyankar, S.D. 1971. On a remarkable new nematode, *Pseudocucullanus tachysuri* gen. et sp. nov. from marine fish of India and *Neocucullanellus yamagutii* n. sp. Riv. Parasit. 32: 37-42.
21. Kirmse, P. and H. Ferguson. 1976. Toxoplasma-like organisms as the possible causative agents of a proliferative condition in farmed Turbot (*Scophthalmus maximum*). In Page: Wildlife Diseases, Plenum, New York, 561-564.
22. Laird, M. 1956. Aspects of Fish Parasitology. Proc. 2 Symp. Malayan Soc. 46-54.
23. Lavier, G. 1938. Sur un protophyte parasite intestinal de poisson marin. Ann. paras. 16: 259-264.
24. Lom, J. 1970. Protozoa causing diseases in marine fishes. In S.F. Snieszko: A Symposium on Diseases of Fishes and Shellfishes. Am. Fish. Soc. Spec. Publ. 5: 101-123.
25. Lom, J. and R.F. Nigrelli. 1970. *Brooklynella hostilis* n. g., n. sp., A Pathogenic Cyrtophorine Ciliate in Marine Fishes. J. Protozool. 17: 224-232.
26. Mac Cosker, J.E. and R.F. Nigrelli. 1971. New Records of Lymphocystis Disease in Four Eastern Pacific Fish Species. J. Fish. Res. Bd. Canada. 28: 1809-1810.
27. Mac Kenzie, K. 1969. *Scyphidia* (*Gerda*) *adunconucleata* n. sp. and *Trichodina borealis* (Protozoa, Ciliata) from Young Plaice in Scottish Waters. J. Fish. Biol. 1: 239-247.
28. Mac Millen, S. and D.S. Kishner. 1959. *Mycobacterium marinum* Bact. Proc. 31.
29. Mann, H. 1970. Copepoda and Isopoda as parasites of marine fishes. In S.F. Snieszko: A Symposium on Diseases of Fishes and Shellfishes. Am. Fish. Soc. Spec. Publ. 5: 177-189.

30. Margolis, L. 1970. Nematode diseases of marine fishes. In: S.F. Snieszko: A Symposium on Diseases of Fishes and Shellfishes. Am. Fish. Soc. Spec. Publ. 5: 190-208.
31. Mawdesley-Thomas, L.E. 1971. Neoplasia in Fish: A Review Curr. Topics comp. Pathob. 1: 87-170.
32. Moevus, L. 1963. Studies on a marine parasitic ciliate as a potential virus vector. Symp. Marine Microbiol. Springfield III.
33. Moevus-Kobb, L. 1965. Studies with IPN virus in marine hosts. Ann. N.Y. Ac. Sci. 126: 328-342.
34. Nigrelli, R.F. 1936. The morphology, cytology and life history of *Oodinium ocellatum*, a dinoflagellate parasite on marine fishes. Zoologica 21: 129-164.
35. Nigrelli, R.F. 1943. Causes of Diseases and Death of Fishes in Captivity. Zoologica 28: 203-216.
36. Nigrelli, R.F. and G.D. Ruggieri. 1966. Enzootics in the New York Aquarium caused by *Cryptocaryon irritans*, a histophagous ciliate in the skin, eyes and gills of marine fishes. Zoologica 51: 97-102.
37. Nigrelli, R.F. and G.M. Smith. 1939. Studies on lymphocystis disease in the orange filefish, *Ceratacanthus schoepfii* from Sandy Hook Bay, N.J. Zoologica 24: 255-264.
38. Nigrelli, R.F. and H. Vogel. 1963. Spontaneous tuberculosis in fishes and in other cold-blooded vertebrates, with special reference to *Mycobacterium fortuitum* from fish and human lesions. Zoologica 48: 131-144.
39. Ollenschlager, B. 1975. Schmerzausschaltung bei Fischen. Berl. Munch. Tierarztl. Wchschr. 88: 302-303.
40. Oppenheimer, C.H. and G.L. Kesteven. 1953. Disease as a factor in natural mortality of marine fish. Fish Bull. FAO 6: 215-222.
41. Peters, G.L. 1975. Seasonal fluctuations in the incidence of epidermal papillomas of the European eel, *Anguilla anguilla*. J. Fish. Biol. 7: 415-422.
42. Peters, N., G. Peters and G. Bresching. 1972. Redifferenzierung und Wachstumshemmung von epidermalen Tumoren des europaischen Aals unter Einwirkung von Chininsulfat. Arch. Fish. Wiss. 23: 47-63.
43. Quignard, J.P. 1963. Rapport entre la presence d'une "gibbosite frontale" chez les Labridae (Poissons, Teleosteens) et le parasite *Leposphilus labrei* (Copepoda Phylichthyidae). Ann. Paras. 43: 51-57.

44. Raabe, H. 1936. Etudes de microorganismes parasites des poissons de mer I. *Nosema ovoideum* Thel. dans le foie des rougets. Bull. Inst. Oceanogr. Monaco 696: 1-2.
45. Raabe, H. 1937. Etudes de microorganismes parasites des poissons de mer II. *Thalamoebella parasitica* n. g., n. sp. Bull. Inst. Oceanogr. Monaco 767: 1-16.
46. Raabe, H. 1940. Etudes de microorganismes parasites des poissons de mer III. *Leucosphaera oxneri* n. g. n. sp., algue provoquant les "points blancs" sur la peau des poissons. Bull. Inst. Oceanogr. Monaco 785: 1-11.
47. Reichenbach-Klinke, H.-H. 1955. Fensterartige Kiemendeckeldefekte beim Seehecht (*Merluccius merluccius*). Mitt. Mus. Aschaffenburg 55-58.
48. Reichenbach-Klinke, H.-H. 1956. Augenschaden bei Meeresfischen durch den Pilz *Ichthyosporidium hoferi* und Bemerkungen zu seiner Verbreitung bei Mittelmeerfischen. Publ. Staz. Zool. Napoli 29: 22-32.
49. Reichenbach-Klinke, H.-H. 1956. Ueber einige bisher unbekannte Hyphomyceten bei verschiedenen Susswasserund Meeresfischen. Mycopath. Mycol. appl. 7: 333-347.
50. Reichenbach-Klinke, H.-H. 1957. Vorlaufige Mitteilung uber die Parasiten der Fische des Golfs von Neapel. Pubbl. Staz. Zool. Napoli 30: 115-126.
51. Reichenbach-Klinke, H.-H. 1966. Krankheiten der Aquarienfische. 2. Aufl., Kernen Stuttgart.
52. Reichenbach-Klinke, H.-H. 1966. Krankheiten und Schadigungen der Fische. Fischer Stuttgart.
53. Reichenbach-Klinke, H.-H. 1970. Vorlaufige Mitteilung und Neubeschreibung einer parasitaren Blastodiniale (Dinoflagellata) Bei Susswasserfischen. Z. Fischerei NF 18: 289-297.
54. Riddell, W. and D.M. Alexander. 1911. Note on an ulcerative disease of the plaice. Prov. Liverp. Biol. Soc. 26: 155-161.
55. Roberts, R.J. 1976. Experimental Pathogenesis of Lymphocystis in the Plaice (*Pleuronectes platessa*). In Page: Wildlife Diseases. Plenum, New York 431-411.
56. Russell, F.S. 1923. A new species of *Caligus* from Egypt, *Caligus pageti* sp. n. Ann. Mag. Nat. Hist. 15: 611-618.
57. Schlumberger, H.G. and B. Lucke. 1948. Tumors of Fishes, Amphibians and Reptiles. Cancer Res. 8: 657-754.
58. Schubert, G. 1969. Exophthalmus caused by thyroid tissue in the choroid layer of the eye in *Coris gaimard*. Bull. Wildlife Dis. Ass. 5: 113.

59. Schubert, V., V. Sprague and R. Reinboth. 1975. Observations on a New Species of *Unicapsula* (Myxosporida) in the Fish *Maena smaris* by Conventional and Electronmicroscopy. Z. Parasitenk. 46: 245-252.
60. Shotts, E.B. and S.F. Snieszo. 1976. Selected Bacterial Fish Diseases. In Page: Wildlife Diseases III. Int. Wildlife.
61. Sikama, Y. 1961. On a new species of *Ichthyophthirius* found in marine fishes. Science Report. Yokosuka City, Mus. 6: 65-70.
62. Sindermann, C.J. 1966. Diseases of Marine Fishes, T.F.H. Publications, Neptune City, N.J.
63. Sindermann, C. and A. Rosenfield. 1954. Diseases of Fishes of the Western North Atlantic. I. Diseases of the sea herring (*Clupea harengus*), Dep. Sea & Shore Fish. Augusta, Maine.
64. Sproston, N.G. 1946. A synopsis of the monogenetic trematodes. Trans. Zool. Soc. London, 25: 185-600.
65. Srivastava, L.P. 1966. Three new leeches (Piscicolidae) from marine shore fishes (Cottidae) in British waters. J. Zool. London 150: 297-318.
66. Tsutsumi, T., A. Murata and M. Murața. 1963. Studien unber die Ausrottung der Weissfleckenkrankheit bei Seefischen. Dobutsuen Suiz. Zassli 5: 35-44.
67. Valentine, D.W. 1975. Skeletal anomalies in Marine Teleosts. In Ribelin & Migaki: The Pathology of Fishes. Wisconsin Press, Madison/London, 695-718.
68. Wells, N.A. and C.E. ZoBell. *Achromobacter ichthyodermis* n. sp., the etiological agent of an infectious dermatitis of certain marine fishes. Proc. Nat. Ac. Sci. 20: 123-126.
69. Wodjanizkii, W.A., W.N. Grese, M.A. Dolgopolskaja, and E.W. Pawlowa. 1968. Parasity morskich shiwotnych. Heft 14 von Biologija Morja. Ak. Nauk Ukrain. SSR Kiew.
70. Wossner, H. 1974. Written communication.
71. Wunder, W. 1962. *Nerocila orbignyi*, ein proterandrischer Hermaphrodit und parasitischer Isopode auf *Tilapia galilaea* im See Borullus in Agypten. Verh. Dtsch. Zool. Ges. Saarbrucken 1961: 140-151.
72. Yamaguti, S. 1963. Systema helminthum. Interscience Publ., New York, London.
73. Yamaguti, S. 1968. Monogenetic trematodes of Hawaiian fishes. Honolulu, Univ. Hawaii Press.

Index

(Entries set in **bold** face denote illustrations.)

The Famous
Pacific Marine Fishes Series

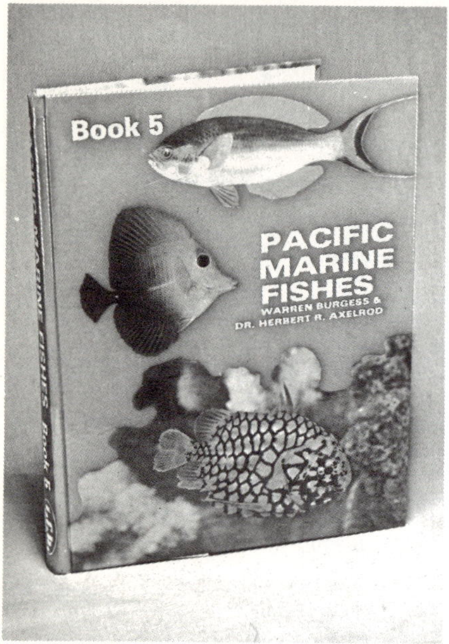

PACIFIC MARINE FISHES, Book 1
(Coastal waters of southern Japan and the Ryukyu Islands.) Text covers entirely different group of families from Book 2. *TFH PS-697*

PACIFIC MARINE FISHES, Book 2
(Coastal waters of southern Japan and the Ryukyu Islands.) Text covers entirely different group of families from Book 1. *TFH PS-699*

PACIFIC MARINE FISHES, Book 3
(Covers Maldive Islands to Mombasa in East Africa.) *TFH PS-719*

PACIFIC MARINE FISHES, Book 4
(Taiwan and adjacent waters.) Text covers entirely different group of families from book 5. *TFH PS-720*

PACIFIC MARINE FISHES, Book 5
(Taiwan and adjacent waters.) Text covers entirely different group of families from Book 4. *TFH PS-721*

PACIFIC MARINE FISHES, Book 6
(Melanesia) *TFH PS-722*

PACIFIC MARINE FISHES, Book 7
(Great Barrier Reef) *TFH PS-723*

PACIFIC MARINE FISHES Books 8 through 12 will cover different geographical areas, as follows: Book 8, Tasman Sea; Book 9, Hawaii; Book 10, Western Americas; Book 11, Red Sea; Book 12, Western Australia.

Here is a series of books that are of great interest and high value to marine hobbyists. They talk about and show—almost entirely in beautiful true-to-life big full color illustrations—some of the most interesting and dazzlingly colorful fishes in the world. Each book in the series (currently seven books are available, with five additional books planned) is big (8½ x 11", over 270 pages), expensively produced and lavishly colorful. Each is accompanied by an eye-opening text that probes the fascinating highlights of the fish families covered; the text is up to date and painstakingly accurate, yet easy and enjoyable to read. Each book is completely indexed and contains about 400 color photos. The famous *Pacific Marine Fishes* series has captivated marine hobbyists because of the books' beauty and usefulness in identifying and learning about saltwater species, especially those that have never been photographed before, even though they're perfect for marine aquaria. Make an investment in reading pleasure by getting your first book today—you'll soon want the others.

Each book in the series is priced at $20, available at pet shops and book stores everywhere.

T.F.H. Publications, Inc.

P.O. Box 27 • Neptune, NJ 07753